T0109127

DO YOU DARE?

65 SEX GAMES TO HEAT UP YOUR SEX LIFE

DO YOU DARE?

65 SEX GAMES TO HEAT UP YOUR SEX LIFE

TINA ROBBINS

TRANSLATED BY DON MCGINNIS

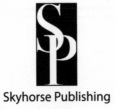

Skyhorse Publishing

Many of the activities described in this book are by their very nature daring, outrageous, and sometimes even illegal and potentially hazardous. They are suggested only for consenting adults who understand that they assume sole responsibility for their own actions and safety, and for any resulting professional or legal consequences. The information and suggestions in this book cannot replace sound judgment and good decision-making. Further, no one should take any action or participate in any activity, if he or she feels at all uncomfortable or uncertain about the cicumstances or risks.

Original title: SEXO PARA MUJERES ATREVIDAS
© 2013 Editorial Océano, S.L. (Barcelona, Spain)

All rights reserved. No part of this publication may be reproduced or stored in a retrieval system or transmitted in any form or by any means, whether electronic, mechanical, photocopying, recording or other kind, without the prior permission in writing by the owners.

English translation © 2016 by Skyhorse Publishing

All rights reserved. No part of this book may be reproduced in any manner without the express written consent of the publisher, except in the case of brief excerpts in critical reviews or articles. All inquiries should be addressed to Skyhorse Publishing, 307 West 36th Street, 11th Floor, New York, NY 10018.

Skyhorse Publishing books may be purchased in bulk at special discounts for sales promotion, corporate gifts, fund-raising, or educational purposes. Special editions can also be created to specifications. For details, contact the Special Sales Department, Skyhorse Publishing, 307 West 36th Street, 11th Floor, New York, NY 10018 or info@skyhorsepublishing.com.

Skyhorse® and Skyhorse Publishing® are registered trademarks of Skyhorse Publishing, Inc.®, a Delaware corporation.

Visit our website at www.skyhorsepublishing.com.

10 9 8 7 6 5 4 3 2 1

Library of Congress Cataloging-in-Publication Data is available on file.

Cover design by Qualcom Designs
Cover photo credit Thinkstock

ISBN: 978-1-63450-344-0
Ebook ISBN 978-1-63450-906-0

Printed in the United States of America

Contents

I Was a Vanilla Lover. 9

The Pleasure of the Forbidden 13

Out with Clichés. 19

Switch Gears. 21

The Three Zones. 23

Dos and Don'ts of a Daring Lover. 25

Where Do I Start?. 31

BDSM, to the Limit 33
   Dominant or Submissive. 34
   Would You Rather Be a Switch? 36
   Safety Before All Else 37

65 Games to the Limit. 39
   1. Blindfolded 39
   2. No Escape 41

3. Knots of Pleasure 42
4. Bondage Positions 43
5. Swinging 44
6. Make Me Submit 45
7. Step Hard 47
8. Dressed for the Occasion 48
9. You've Been Bad 49
10. Dinner Is Served 50
11. Trying Aphrodisiacs 51
12. Burning Sessions 52
13. My Slave's Collar 53
14. Total Control 54
15. My Master's Briefcase 55
16. Look at Me, Look at You 56
17. Will You Climb on My Swing? 57
18. Punish Me, Darling 60
19. Strong Emotions 61
20. Eat Me 62
21. Tell Me 62
22. Wireless Sex 63
23. Sexting: Look How Hot I Am! 64
24. "Oral" Sex 65
25. Pegging: Do You Dare? 65
26. Anal Pleasure 66
27. The Contract 66
28. Here and Now 69
29. Warming the Engines 70
30. Very Intimate Jewelry 72
31. To the Water! 72
32. Get Naked for Me 73
33. Recording 74
34. Shall We Meet? 75
35. In a Hairy 76
36. The Box of Desires 77
37. Sex Is an Affair for Two . . . or Three 79

38. A Tantric Night 81
39. The Foolproof Weapon 83
40. Cover Your Legs 84
41. Free Your Imagination. 85
42. A Sensual Piercing. 87
43. You're Welcome. 88
44. The Forbidden Zone 90
45. Submissive Fellatio 92
46. The Warrior's Rest. 93
47. Online Inspiration. 95
48. A Different Kind of Masturbation. 96
49. A Burlesque Night. 97
50. Sweet Veneration. 98
51. Non-Consensual Sex. 99
52. Lovers with a Sweet Tooth. 100
53. Chilling 102
54. This Is Good for 102
55. Please, Go On!. 103
56. A Good Ally 105
57. Can I Have Your Belt? 106
58. Fortune Cookies 107
59. By the Hair. 109
60. Facefuck: Pure Domination 110
61. Bare Your Teeth 111
62. Endless Torture 112
63. Let's Do 69. 113
64. Let's Play!. 114
65. Lap Dance: Melt Him with Pleasure 115

Glossary 117

I Was a Vanilla Lover

I'll confess something to you: a few years ago, just before I moved to Germany for work reasons, I met a very special person. I don't like to encourage stereotypes, but Erik was a typical Nordic man: tall, strong, with dark blue eyes, a straight beard, and blond, trimmed hair. I needed a tutor to help me perfect my German, and the language school gave me his contact information. We ended up in a café in town. I remember thinking at first that he seemed somewhat abrupt and distant. But there was something about that man that made me feel safe, and we eventually decided to have three classes at home every week until I moved.

Spending so much time talking caused our relationship to eventually become something more personal. There was barely a month left before the move when, one afternoon, we started talking about our personal lives. At the time, I was single and tended to have brief and sporadic relationships. Our chat lengthened, and it became dark before we knew it. "Why don't you stay for dinner?" I asked, convinced that he would decline.

After giving me a deep, calm look, he sighed and offered to cook me a vegetable stew from his country with his grandmother's "secret" touch. We opened a bottle of white wine and had a delightful evening. By morning, Erik was sleeping naked in my bed. The sun was shining in through the window, defining his muscular back. I slid my hand under the cover, ran my fingers down his spine, and gently caressed his glutes. Erik turned over, leaving his hard member exposed, and I took advantage of this generous "offer." After two orgasms, practically one after the other, I looked, horrified, at the clock and ran to work. With no time to shower, his smell stayed with me for the whole day. I knew that this was a passing fling with nowhere to go. In barely a month, I would be a thousand miles away and it wasn't worth it to string him along. We kept going with the lessons, and there were several more nights of sex, each one more intense and unrestrained. We both knew that this had an expiration date, and so we let ourselves get carried away.

In bed, Erik was active; as a lover, he had inexhaustible resources.

"Would you like to stop being a vanilla lover?" he asked me one night, while showing me a length of rope. I confess, that scared me a bit.

"What do you mean? You don't like how sweet I am?" I joked, to disguise my trepidation.

"Imagine you walk into a luxurious ice cream shop, brimming with flavors, colors, and textures. You can ask for whatever you want, experiment, mix, and taste. But you always end up asking for vanilla ice cream. Sex is that ice cream shop. It offers everything you could want to try. You can keep asking for the usual, and be conventional and boring, or you can open yourself up to new sensations and experiences that you've never tried before. Do you dare?" he whispered in my ear while gently tying my wrists.

After that night, I voluntarily became Erik's slave. Submissive and obedient, I signed a sex contract that forced me to follow his every order, accept his punishments, and to be always available for my master's cravings and sexual requirements. Roleplaying, facesitting, spanking, swapping partners, bondage . . . Each night I submerged myself in an exciting universe of luxury and pleasure. Never before had I experienced orgasms this long and intense, I assure you. I was exhausted, but I wished for every night to come sooner so I could fulfill the requirements set out in my sex contract.

This is how the days passed until I finally had to leave for my new job and break off our relationship. I've never heard from him again, but I preserve intact memories of every single moment I shared with this singular lover.

I still like vanilla ice cream, but I've learned to mix flavors, try new sensations, and make my fantasies a reality, without complications, prejudices, or fears.

I invite you to my ice cream shop: would you like to come in?

The Pleasure of the Forbidden

Millions of women around the world have experienced an intimate and delicious revolution with the arrival in bookstores of *Fifty Shades of Grey*. The successful trilogy by British author E. L. James (*Fifty Shades of Grey*, *Fifty Shades Darker*, and *Fifty Shades Freed*) has broken, once and for all, the sexual monotony of many people. Its pages invite you to follow your instincts, shed your shame, and go beyond the limits of pleasure by emulating the intense relationship between its protagonists, the seductive millionaire, Christian Grey, and his lover, the young college student, Anastasia Steele. Reading it has made women of all ages fantasize and—why not?—put the exciting scenes of the book into practice. These scenes introduce the reader to the world of sadomasochism through very descriptive, sensual, and unconventional sex.

New sensations and new lifestyles are born in the most sexual and active organ: our brain. Pleasure, arousal, kink, and stimulation are processes that begin inside the brain and determine our behavior and manner of reacting during intimate relations. Sex would be nothing without the presence of an erotic imagination, fantasies, and seduction. And beyond the same old bodily pleasure that we feel when being physically stimulated in certain parts of our anatomy, there is an equally, or even more, important mental erotic pleasure present in our intimate relations. This is experienced through feelings, images in our mind, and physical, sensual contact (although it may be felt without this).

Generally, this mental pleasure is more commonly found in the female sexual experience, which is personally linked to memories, fantasies, dreams, and sensations bound to emotions.

Although we all fantasize, the female mind tends to fantasize about the entire history surrounding the sexual act, while the male mind focuses more on the act itself. However, regardless of the recurring theme, we do this very often: up to 20 percent of women and 55 percent of men have sexual fantasies once a day. Curiously, the practice of "forbidden" sexual relationships (those that we would never be able to actually go through with) is one of the most common fantasies of women, much more so than in men. The practice of sadomasochistic relationships and having sex with one or several strangers tends to be a more frequent fantasy among women. Fantasizing about it during the act of sex can be very pleasurable. "Entertaining ourselves with this type of thinking is not only a good way of arousing ourselves those times when mere contact is insufficient, but it is also an excellent conduit for predisposing ourselves towards sex, increasing desire and pleasure, and thus increasing the intensity of our orgasms," explains therapeutic psychologist Julia Hernández. Fantasizing about high-voltage situations that are different, unique, or strange allows us to amplify our sexual repertoire and enjoy our intimate relations without taboo or feelings of guilt. Those images, those dreams or fantasies, may easily become reality. It is only a question of resolving ourselves and taking the leap, daring to experiment with new sensations, and experiencing sex in new ways. Transgressing, being surprised, trying different positions, and trying BDSM are really efficient techniques for increasing sexual desire and amplifying the frequency and intensity of orgasms. Besides, sexual fantasies help to increase self-esteem and personal appeal, enhance interest and sexual desire, satisfy curiosity, and allow us to rehearse real-life encounters and reduce stressful situations, worrying, and anxiety.

Cataloging sexual fantasies is as complicated as trying to impose limits and labels on imagination. Generally, sexual fantasies are considered to be any type of image or thought that, for that specific person, holds some sexual or erotic meaning. Even so, most fantasies can be placed into five large categories: loving/romantic, homosexual, sadomasochistic, force, and domination/submission.

Among the most common images in our subconscious, we may find:

- **The forbidden or never experienced.** Images of sex in public places or prostitution, which we tend to use in order to defeat routine and monotony in our intimate relationships.

- **Switching partners.** Imagining that we are having sexual relations with someone other than our partner (and usually someone close to us) is one of the most common fantasies among both genders.

- **Group sex.** Orgies, or relationships with more than one person of the same or different sex, fall into this category.

- **Sadomasochism.** Fantasies that feature pain or physical strength.

- **Rape.** Situations of forced sex in which we take the role of the person who rapes or the one who is raped.

What do you fantasize about?

Written in 1988, the so-called "Wilson's Sex Fantasy Questionnaire (SFQ)" is an efficient scale that deeply analyzes the kind of sexual daydreams that we have, as well as our preferences when imagining intimate encounters outside of the routine and habitual.

Each fantasy should be scored from 0 to 3, according to the frequency in which we have them: 0 being never, 1 being rarely, 2 being sometimes, and 3 being often.

1. Taking part in an orgy.
2. Homosexual acts.
3. Switching partners.
4. Promiscuity.
5. Sex with two other people.
6. Sex with someone of a different race.
7. Sex with a loved one.
8. Having intimate relations with someone you know, but who you have not had sexual encounters with.
9. Active oral sex.
10. Having sex outside of the bedroom (in the kitchen, for example).
11. Being stripped.
12. Being masturbated by your partner.
13. Observing the sexual act of others.
14. Having sex with someone dressed in leather or latex.
15. Watching obscene images or movies.
16. Using stimulating objects (vibrators, for example).
17. Wearing clothes of the opposite gender.
18. Being whipped or struck.
19. Tying someone up.
20. Being tied up.
21. Showing off provocatively.
22. Forcing someone to do something.
23. Being forced to do something.

Where does feminine pleasure reside?

In 2001, investigators from Rutgers University, under the leadership of scientist Barry Komisaruk, traced the first mental map of female pleasure, which supplied valuable information about the localization of the sensory areas of the female anatomy. Through magnetic resonance imaging techniques, the team deeply analyzed the sensory responses of several women during different phases of self-stimulation.

The study managed to show, for the first time, that stimulation of the vagina, the uterine wall, and the clitoris activates three different and separate sites in the sensory cortex, with particularly intense activity centered around the uterus and clitoris.

Due to this, Komisaruk's work puts to the test the well-propagated theory that argues that women who obtain pleasure from vaginal stimulation do so only because the clitoris is being indirectly stimulated.

Out with Clichés

During a recent study on sexuality that took place in Great Britain, almost 80 percent of women said that their sex life was at its best once they were beyond their forties. This is because sex is ageless, and it is time to get rid of the absurd sexual clichés that would say otherwise. Sex is good at any age, and especially during the adult years, when men and women may enjoy their sexuality more, without worrying about prejudices or social norms.

Who said that menopause spells the end of sexual relationships for women? Women's pleasure, fun, kinkiness, and desire do not magically disappear, nor are they prevented from having gratifying intimate relationships, no matter how many years go by.

What is really important, more than the hormonal imbalances that a woman (or a man) may experience after a certain age, is to learn to get rid of the routine and create new experiences, games, and moments that will keep our sexual desires in good shape. This turns out to be easy since, after a certain age, duties have been done and a certain sentimental, economic, and work stability allows for enough serenity to develop the sexual facets, alone as much as with a partner. As you know, experience counts.

After a certain age, our physical appearance is not the same as it was twenty years ago. It is time to naturally accept the changes, embrace them, and use them in our favor to experience the most complete and prejudice-free sexuality possible. This will help us to speak sincerely and openly with our partner, express our desires, and suggest introducing new techniques, games, and toys to our sex life so we may live out our relationships with bonus intensity, desire, and pleasure.

Switch Gears

Let's speak frankly: we all have sexual fantasies that we would be excited to make a reality. There is nothing better for enjoying a healthy, passion-filled sex life than letting your imagination fly and realizing that strong, visceral, and rough sex is also an option to keep in mind.

Throughout my career as a speaker on sexual matters, I've attended innumerable talks, debates, and roundtables where attendees have openly talked about their intimate tendencies, fantasies, desires, and lifestyles. I can assure you that we still have a long way to go before we fully enjoy sex. There are too many lines still to cross; there is a lack of communication and far too many taboos.

What if whips get me excited? Am I weird if I like rough sex? Is it strange to make a video recording when I make love to my partner? We are in the twenty-first century and we still let ourselves be swayed by clichés and prejudices when it comes time to get in bed with someone. What if we just let ourselves go once and for all? More than one woman has confessed to me that she feels she has not completely let go during her sexual relations. There is always something that blocks her and keeps her from intensely feeling and experimenting. Let's see . . . What is sex for, if not to relax and let yourself be taken away by desire and enjoyment? I know of too many cases in which a couple's sex life ends up a regular and boring routine. Setting aside one day a week for sex, forgetting to take the initiative in bed, always using the same techniques, or using them in the same order are errors that many couples tend to make in their intimate relationships. Sex is imagination, it is change, it is surprise. Letting yourself go always brings better results than rigid, programmed relations. One day, you might try a session of strokes and massages. Another night, dare to try out some different positions or experiment in different parts of the home, such as the bathroom, the terrace, or on the kitchen table.

The key lies in finding all the new ingredients that will spice up your relations and keep you far away from routine. Working, studying, taking the kids to school, making dinner—these are things that can become tedious, but sex never should. Woody Allen said that it was the most fun you could have without laughing, so start doing it and switch gears.

The Three Zones

We all remember that daring lover or that special night when we had sex using positions, games, or an intensity that was beyond ordinary. In life, there are always frontiers that we must cross, and limits that, upon exceeding them, provide us with all kinds of sensations (doubt, fear, pleasure, excitement, etc.). The same thing happens with intimate relationships. Our sexual desires change as we accumulate experience, and as we break limits, taboos, and prejudices. While we do this, we are expanding what is known as our "comfort zone," a term that is used in sexology to refer to the ensemble of sexual activities with which we feel most comfortable and, consequently, practice most frequently.

Imagine that comfort zone is like a great round ring that surrounds us. Beyond the border of that ring lies an inhospitable territory, a larger circular area: the learning zone. This is a zone that we occasionally visit, and within which we experience more intense sexual games that we still don't know if we like. When we finally find an experience that we like, and incorporate it into our regular sexual repertoire, we have expanded our comfort zone. Logically, as the years go by and we gather experience, this zone gets bigger and bigger.

One of the goals of this book is for you to dare to enter the so-called "panic or rejection zone." This is the furthest zone away from our comfort zone, and here we may find the sexual experiences that (supposedly) we do not wish to try. What happens is that if we like discovering new sensations, bit by bit the comfort zone will approach this outside area, meaning that we will surely explore it eventually.

Imagination, creativity, communication with a partner, and the desire to try new things and evolve will cause our comfort zone to grow larger and larger. To achieve this, one must fully enjoy a rich sex life full of emotions, experiences, and surprises. I hope you get there.

Dos and Don'ts of a Daring Lover

1. **Do not suppress yourself.** One of the things that most excites men in bed is knowing that they are driving their lover wild. Be aware, though: we are not talking about faking orgasms, exaggerated moaning, or behaving crazily or irrationally. The key is to be natural and show yourself for who you are, without suppressing yourself, concealing feelings, or blocking reactions. In this sense, body language is an excellent tool for showing your lover that you are having a great time. Can you talk dirty? Talking dirty means using words or phrases saturated with eroticism (obscene or not) to kick your relations up a couple of notches. It might seem strange at first, but it is a great tool that will help your lover discover what most excites or upsets you at any given time. Plus, when it comes to BDSM, this becomes a safety measure because it allows you to set a key word that will announce that the line between what is pleasurable and what is uncomfortable or excessively painful is being crossed.

2. **Take the initiative.** Until just recently, it was thought that the man's role was to always take sexual initiative. Fortunately, things have changed and that first step now falls equally to both sexes. Even with this social taboo gone, many women

are still unwilling to guide their own intimate relationships and allow themselves to be led instead. It's not due to laziness or indifference; it is because they aren't daring. Fear of rejection or feeling ridiculous causes them to opt for what is more comfortable—that is, to wait for the other person to take the reins and decide for themselves how relations will play out. Ideally, there should be a certain alternation in the initiative and each partner should be equally capable of taking the lead and letting themselves go. Besides, when it comes to wanting to try more daring sex games, it might be best to take the baton in order to show our partner what we hope to get from this new experience. And don't forget about foreplay. It serves to increase the sexual tension so that orgasms are much more intense and lasting, in both men and women. Contrary to popular opinion, men also require and enjoy foreplay. In fact, the foreplay will make the erection much more firm and the coitus more intense. For women, it will cause the vagina to dilate and lubricate, facilitating penetration and the level of excitement necessary to achieve orgasm. Did you know that the average duration of the sexual act is twenty-two minutes? A bit short, surely. But if you learn to enjoy the foreplay that comes before the main event, you will have much more fun, and your partner will as well. You just need a little bit of inspiration. Keep reading; it's time to try out some games.

3. **Fulfill your fantasies.** Sex is devotion and, as such, it is important to thoroughly know the desires, fantasies, and erotic daydreams of your lover in order to help make them a reality, without shame or doubt. Because of this, I reiterate how important it is that the couple communicate openly and learn to talk about sex without prejudice. Sexual fantasies aren't just an escape from reality; they also stimulate desire for the unreachable.

4. **A good arsenal.** The best way to get started with specific sexual techniques is to incorporate certain toys or sexual elements into our relationships. A simple pair of handcuffs, a small whip, a vibrator, or a pair of latex boots could be an excellent invitation to let our lover know that we want to go further during our relations. Remember that the element of surprise is an infallible aphrodisiac, and very exciting. Without warning, casually incorporate one of these toys in the midst of your relations and you'll see how you will add an unexpected and enjoyable twist to the proceedings. Erotic jewelry, dildos, flavored condoms, massage oils, masks, anal stimulators, bondage ropes, and swings—throughout this book, we will talk thoroughly about the use and enjoyment of different, surprising sex toys that we may incorporate into our most intimate sessions.

5. **Renew your appetite.** Did you know that our bodies are perfectly prepared to have sex every day? Doing so does not physically weaken us or psychologically wear us down. There is no frequency that is considered "normal" when it comes to sexual relations, but if you want to become a more daring lover, you clearly should start by increasing the frequency of your intimate encounters. Aside from having more opportunities to try out more daring sex games, you will also proportionally increase your sexual desire. That is according to Fisher's Law, which states that the more sexually active a couple is, the more their desire increases. According to the data from a large-scale survey of more than 26,000 people across the world by Harris Interactive, a market research team, on behalf of Durex, the condom manufacturer, the Greek, Brazilians, Russians, and Chinese are the most passionate lovers—up to 80 percent of their populations have sex at least once per week. The list ends with the Japanese and North Americans, who have the least amount of sex.

6. **Think about sex.** It's not enough just to do it. To become a daring lover capable of driving your partner wild, it's important that you get used to always thinking all kinds of sexual thoughts. Don't feel dirty or vulgar doing so. Remember that the brain is the principal erogenous zone. Stimulating it with erotic ideas, techniques, and situations is the best way to keep your libido at its best and to be fully ready when it comes time to put it to use.

7. **Two is better than one.** Fortunately, the female body is blessed with the ability to have multiple orgasms. Our sexual response cycle, in the final stage, does not go through a refractory period. This allows us to have multiple orgasms during sexual relations. With this in mind, don't settle for a single climax, and search for ways to have new orgasms.

8. **Get in shape.** Abdominals, glutes, biceps . . . To increase your sexual stamina, it's necessary to exercise all your muscles to keep them in good shape and ready to work at their full potential. And don't forget to strengthen your pelvic muscles by regularly doing Kegel exercises. These consist of contracting and relaxing the pubococcygeus muscle repeatedly with the goal of increasing their resistance and tonicity. It is recommended to start gradually (about fifty contractions a day) and to increase the repetitions over time until you reach two hundred daily. Since it simply consists of squeezing and relaxing the muscle (as if you were trying to keep from having to pee), the exercise can be done at any time or in any place (watching television, sitting in the office, on the subway, etc.). If you prefer, there are physical therapists that specialize in the pelvic floor who can help you keep your so-called "pleasure muscles" in shape. Another way of strengthening this area involves using Ben Wa balls. Also known as Burmese bells, they are two spheres that contain a smaller sphere inside, linked together by a length of cord, that are introduced into

the vagina. When the woman moves or walks, the balls knock into each other, providing a soft and pleasant stimulation.

9. **Do you know your hot spots?** Aside from the common erogenous zones located on the sex organs, each person has their own areas of pleasure. Spread throughout the whole body, these are areas where there is a greater number of nerve endings. When adequately stimulated, they send torrents of pleasurable sensations and sexual arousal to the brain. These responses are not automatic in every case, nor are they identical from person to person. To help you find your hot spots, you can take the following test with your partner. It consists of grading the amount of pleasure you feel when stroked, kissed, or stimulated on different parts of your body. You'll find out some interesting things that you can use during your next sexual encounter.

Lips	0 1 2 3 4	Armpits	0 1 2 3 4
Face	0 1 2 3 4	Arms	0 1 2 3 4
Ears	0 1 2 3 4	Hands	0 1 2 3 4
Neck	0 1 2 3 4	Thighs	0 1 2 3 4
Chest	0 1 2 3 4	Back	0 1 2 3 4
Nipples	0 1 2 3 4	Glutes	0 1 2 3 4

Feet	0 1 2 3 4	**Scoring:**
Fingers	0 1 2 3 4	Uncomfortable = 0
Abdomen	0 1 2 3 4	No feeling = 1
Belly button	0 1 2 3 4	Somewhat pleasurable = 2
Groin	0 1 2 3 4	Very pleasurable = 3
Nape of the neck	0 1 2 3 4	Orgasmic = 4
Shoulders	0 1 2 3 4	
Hair	0 1 2 3 4	
Skin	0 1 2 3 4	

When you find your body's most erogenous zones, remember that no one is a mind-reader, so it is most important to be open and communicative with your partner.

10. **Dare!** Every single one of the sexual tips in this book will require a bit of daring. So take the leap and experiment, investigate, ask, and test. Increase your sexual confidence, take the reins of your pleasure, and launch yourself into discovering the new limits of your sexual relations. Stop and think for a moment: what is the most daring thing you've ever tried in bed? If you've never gone further than trying out a couple of positions, a bit of oral sex, or a couple of little toys, it's time to increase the intensity and variety of your intimate encounters if you don't want to fall into routine and kill your partner with boredom. Now, you want to kill him with pleasure!

Where Do I Start?

Communication is very important in maintaining a sex life that is complete, exciting, and fun. Because that's what it's all about, right? Enjoying sex necessitates staying far away from routines and not allowing any attitudes or preferences that could plunge the relationship into monotony. Mind you, it might be the case that one of you might be more active or curious when it comes to trying new things. They key is not to be timid or restrained when sharing those interests with your partner. For example, if BDSM piques our curiosity, we can bring the topic up bit by bit and see how our partner reacts. Watching movies like *The Ages of Lulu* or others that feature things we would like to try is a good start in hinting to our partner.

A bit of literature

To get started with the philosophy of BDSM games and techniques, there is an extensive and suggestive catalog of erotic literature about it. Here are some of the recommended titles:

- *Story of O*, by Pauline Réage (1954)
- *Nine and a Half Weeks*, by Elizabeth McNeil (1978)
- *The Ties That Bind*, by Vanessa Duriès (1993)
- *Submission: a Novel*, by Marthe Blau (2002)

Aside from that specific topic, there are also other stimulating pieces of literature you might share with your partner. Some suggestions:

- *Lady Chatterley's Lover*, by D. H. Lawrence (1928)
- *Lolita*, by Vladimir Nabokov (1955)
- *Fear of Flying*, by Erica Jong (1973)
- *Delta of Venus*, by Anaïs Nin (1978)

"You see, darling? Wouldn't you like to try that sometime . . . ?" you can ask him. It will get him thinking. It goes without saying that reading the trilogy by E. L. James together could be very inspiring (and exciting, I assure you).

BDSM, to the Limit

BDSM is an acronym, the letters of which mean bondage, discipline and domination, submission and sadism, and masochism. It encompasses a number of techniques and sexual hobbies that have one element in common: the participants build, voluntarily and consensually, a relationship in which one of them takes on the role of the dominant, or active, party, while the other is passive or submissive.

Between partners, the practice becomes more and more extensive thanks to the infinite possibilities that can be naturally interspersed among all the other sex games. This prevents the couple from falling into a routine and brings more fun and intense excitement to the relationship.

Did you know?

July 24 is celebrated around the world as the International BDSM Day—a date that was deliberately chosen because it references the submissiveness shown to the master twenty-four hours a day, seven days a week. This is one of the more extreme practices in this type of relationship, where the partners extend their roles to apply during all hours of the day, as if they were permanently living in the created situation. This practice receives the name of 24/7, or TPE (Total Power Exchange), and can be exciting to try out on vacations, for example, when the couple has more time at their disposal.

It may seem rare, but the truth is that many couples incorporate some elements of BDSM into their sex lives. This could mean using tie-downs with handkerchiefs or handcuffs, or other things like pinching, biting, or scratching the partner during relations. In fact, according to a recent survey done in Spain, about 20 percent of the people interviewed admitted to having tried some form of BDSM, and almost 50 percent had fantasized about possibly trying it.

Dominant or Submissive

Before initiating yourself into BDSM's exciting acts of intense and non-conventional sex, you should decide which role you want to play during your intimate encounters. Essentially, you may choose the dominant or submissive role. The dominant is the person who takes initiative and control at all times, while the submissive person limits themselves to receiving pleasure by submitting their will to the orders and requirements of the dominant person.

If you chose the dominant role, keep in mind that this does not mean simply giving random orders. The charm of this role lies in getting the submissive person to find pleasure in being dominated. During this type of intense experience, pain and pleasure are intimately linked. A good master, with a personality that is strong and determined yet serene and protective, can make these two things indistinguishable, provoking very exciting sensations.

As a lover, the dominant person should show affection, attentiveness, support, and tenderness whenever the situation calls for it. Many think that the relationship between the dominant and the submissive is based on a show of strength and control. Nothing could be further from the truth. This is a consensual relationship that, as such, should not be harmful to the submissive party.

The submissive person, in their role, must always follow the orders and indications of their master, although they may also be active and give opinions, share, and on occasion even guide the activities. Experts in this practice consider that the main role of the submissive person is to give their master pleasure, forgetting about their own—not because they are afraid, or being punished or rewarded, but because they want their master to be happy and do not wish to displease them by any means.

When opting for the role of master/dominant, the first step is to choose the type of domination you wish to exercise. This could be:

- **Physical.** This is domination that includes the use of elements such as ropes, handcuffs, crops, and whips. These may accompany the restriction of movement of the person being submitted. This practice requires a good amount of control over the situation at all times to avoid accidents or misunderstandings. We will soon go over the importance of having a key safety word agreed upon by both lovers that can be used in case the situation spirals out of control or becomes excessively painful or uncomfortable for the submissive person. Remember that communication between partners is very important for this kind of practice.

- **Verbal.** This is the kind of domination that is ideal for starting with BDSM. This is a less direct technique than physical domination and is based on using words or phrases to order the submissive person to obey whatever the master/dominant's will.

What kind of dominant do you want to be?

Generally, there are three roles available to the dominant, keeping in mind that their behavior and the actions they demand will depend greatly on their natural state of being. Among the most common, you may choose the role of:

- **Master.** This is the dominant par excellence, whose sense of ownership over their lover is very defined. The master, be they a man or woman, doesn't just limit himself/herself to giving orders, but also worries about their lover, cares for and helps their lover, and is preoccupied at all times with their lover's thoughts and feelings. This is the role adopted by Christian Grey in the famous trilogy by E. L. James.
- **Despot.** This is the role taken by the dominant who puts their own pleasure (especially sexual) above that of their lover. They are not excessively worried about the thoughts or feelings of their partner, never think about their emotions, and demand while giving nothing in return. This is an exciting role to use in the short term, since longer use could end up bothering the person who is subjected to such a selfish character.
- **Devoted.** This is the lightest profile of all. It consists of a dominant who barely dominates and simply receives and accepts the devotion of the submissive person. This docility is ideal when starting out with BDSM relationships, since it is very comfortable for both members of the game: the dominant does not feel that they are excessive in their role, while the submissive doesn't suffer humiliation or punishments that they do not wish for.

Would You Rather Be a Switch?

Depending on the moment in the relationship, you may wish to alternate between the roles of dominant and submissive, which is referred to in the BDSM world as a "switch." Switching roles is actually recommended because it incorporates the element of surprise into the relationship. Each person has their own nature and interprets the roles in their own manner, which undoubtedly keeps routine and boredom at bay. Besides, this alternating can also be used to add sessions of conventional or "vanilla" sex alongside the exciting nights of alternative sex. One might not always be in the mood to engage in sadomasochistic sessions, just as one might get tired of an excessive amount of light, routine sessions. Keep in mind, also, that the dominant role requires the grasp of certain techniques in order to avoid accidents. Because of this, when in a relationship with alternating roles, it is important that both partners have enough experience and control over the situation as well as sufficient skill with the tools that may be used.

Safety Before All Else

The letters SSC (Safe, Sane, and Consensual) stand for the core idea on which every BDSM relationship should be based. This kind of practice should be pleasurable at all times, as much for the master/dominant as for the slave/submissive. To accomplish this, the games should be safe and participants should employ techniques and tools with which they are familiar enough to avoid possible risks.

Sanity is another fundamental component of this kind of activity. It is important at all times to be able to identify the line between reality and fantasy, as well as not interfering with either party's ability to make decisions through the consumption of alcohol or other substances. Finally, the games should always be consensual between both partners, who must agree upon the manner and intensity of the activities that are taking place—an agreement that may be withdrawn at any time, without any imposition. Given that certain BDSM activities may go beyond what is pleasurable at any given point, it is best to agree with your partner on some gesture or key word that will clearly indicate that it is time to stop the game and not continue.

Most intense sexual practices involving aspects of BDSM come with a certain degree of risk, physical as well as emotional. In avoiding unwanted accidents or damage, it is important to take advantage of material resources as well as education and experience to minimize the danger. For example, before jumping into a bondage session, learn the knots involved, as well as how to use the different kinds of ropes and tethers. Or, if you are trying a wax session, you should learn how to manage the different temperatures of the wax to avoid burning your lover's skin.

In any case, you should always have a first-aid kit at hand and avoid any practices you might not be able to manage with precision. At the end of the day, having fun is what matters the most, so it's best to avoid doing anything that will spoil the party.

As far as emotional security is concerned, I reiterate the importance of maintaining open lines of communication with your partner at all times to avoid uncomfortable situations.

65 Games to the Limit

1. Blindfolded

Watching your lover as you make love can be just as exciting as . . .
not seeing him at all. Eyesight is possibly the most erotic sense of all,
but stop for a moment and think about the sensations you might get
from the scent of your partner, the feeling of his skin, the sound of
his panting, or the taste of his lips.

Using all your senses will make your experience in bed much
more intense, but it is also interesting to deprive oneself of some
of them to experience the rest of them with even more intensity. Men are especially visual and get hot from barely glancing
at the curves of their girl, so it might be particularly exciting
to deprive them of this sense and bring a breath of fresh air to
your sex games. Using blindfolds is a very common practice in
domination sex games. Remember that the brain is the most
sensual organ of them all. One excellent way of stimulating it is
to cover the eyes of your lover, forcing them to maximize the use
of the rest of their senses. Without being able to see you, it will
be much easier for them to free their imagination. Besides, this
game depends on your desire to keep them completely at your
disposal and under the control of your movements. To make
the sensations much more intense, you can incorporate some
toys that raise the heat of the moment even more. Go over your

lover's naked body with soft feathers; pinch, lick, and scratch his skin where he least expects it. Brush his penis using different textures, let him "savor" your most erogenous areas, whisper everything you're going to do to him while you tie his hands to the headboard . . .

With his eyes covered, it's much easier to stimulate other senses such as smell or taste. Thus, oral sex can turn into a different and much more exciting experience. Invite your lover to try a "tasting menu," letting him sample all kinds of flavors served on different parts of your body—cream on your nipples, chocolate on your lips, honey on the tips of your fingers, pieces of fruit on your tongue, and shots of tequila served from your navel. Make him try all sorts of mixtures and textures, lovingly make him guess what flavors or parts or your body he is tasting, and subject him to small tortures if he doesn't guess right.

Give your blindfolded lover no respite and gift him with an erotic massage. In this case, your partner's sensations will be much more intense because he won't know where your hands (or your mouth) are going.

When blindfolding your partner, it's important to do it without using too much pressure, being sure that he is able to breathe comfortably at all times. You can use a silk kerchief, a mask, a t-shirt, or a suggestive piece of lingerie.

Hearing is another sense we can stimulate during one of these "blind" sessions. If you have decided to stop being a vanilla lover, take advantage of this moment to bring your lips to his ear and slowly whisper all the things you are going to do to him. This is not the time to be timid. Leave your well-mannered self behind and let loose your daring and vulgar side. Confess to him your sexual fantasies with a sharp tongue. Don't be delicate. Speak clearly and directly. The idea is to light up your lover's imagination with suggestive, unabashed words and phrases.

If you are a little shy, you might have a hard time finding the right words. A bit of music might help you to sink into the moment. Remember that your guy will have his eyes covered and you can employ the element of surprise whenever you want. Here is a suggestive playlist to give your craziest nights a soundtrack:

"Justify My Love," by Madonna
"Believe," by the Chemical Brothers
"Supermassive Black Hole," by Muse
"Where Have You Been," by Rihanna
"Drumming Song," by Florence + the Machine
"Heaven," by Depeche Mode
"Oniria e Insomnia," by Love of Lesbian
"Let's Get It On," by Marvin Gaye
"Playsong," by The Cure
"Varúð," by Sigur Ros
"All Along the Watchtower," by Jimi Hendrix

2. No Escape

I confess that one of my favorite sexual fantasies is for a virile and somewhat rough man to handcuff me to the headboard and submit me to his will. I can already feel a light tingling just writing these lines.

Among my favorite "toys" are handcuffs and shackles. Both are used to immobilize the person, and it is important to keep certain precautions in mind. Generally, they should be made of stainless steel and have a safety feature that can be used to keep the pressure from causing unwanted injuries. When using them, never leave the handcuffed person alone; opt for shorter sessions, and make sure that there is always a set of spare keys on hand. If you wish to go a bit further, most specialized stores have a great variety of immobilizing tools that you can use to fulfill your most exciting fantasies: double handcuffs for the wrists and neck with chains, ankle cuffs, collars and cuffs connected with an adjustable belt to immobilize the hands behind the back, silk and leather-covered handcuffs, etc. I'm melting with pleasure!

3. Knots of Pleasure

Bondage (a word that comes from the word "bind") is an exciting sexual technique that consists of partially or totally immobilizing your lover using ropes. It is a fundamental part of the BDSM philosophy and is closely linked to domination/submission. On one hand, the person being tied up can become very aroused by feeling completely at the disposal of their "captor," and on the other hand, it is sensual knowing that you can do whatever you like to your partner.

We can choose from different kinds of bondage, according to the preference of each party. You might completely bind the body, totally immobilizing the person; you might bind just a specific part (such as the breasts); you could suspend the bound person (only recommended for people who are very experienced with the technique); and you can enhance the session with gags, masks, etc.

A good way to start out with this type of sex game is to opt for some softer, painless versions until you feel more comfortable going to higher levels. You can try positions that allow you to take hold of your partner and limit their movements. For example, penetrating from behind makes it easier to hold the person by the arms and maintain physical contact with them at all times.

It is important to choose ropes that are made with natural fibers, as they are more pleasing to the touch and tend not to cause painful chafing on the skin.

Another interesting option is elastic cords. Made of synthetic rubber and covered in nylon fiber and other materials, they are highly elastic, capable of stretching to three times their length when pulled.

Playing with rope does have its risks. This is why it is important to always have a reliable cutting tool at hand to avoid any accidents that may harm your partner. Medical emergency professionals use special scissors that have a blunt end, allowing one to insert it between the rope or clothing and the skin without causing harm. It would be best to practice with them so that if you need them, you can react quickly and efficiently. Knives and razors are not recommended for cutting rope during a bondage session.

Other safety tips when using bondage:

- Never loop rope (or anything else) around the neck.
- Never leave a bound person alone.
- Minimize the bound person's risk of stumbling or falling.
- Avoid using slipknots or tricky knots.
- Plan short sessions, especially if the person being bound is inexperienced.
- Do not attempt excessively complex knots if you are not sure you can untie them easily and quickly.

4. Bondage Positions

Binding your partner's hands or legs is a very exciting BDSM practice, but it can be a little tricky finding the ideal position to comfortably enjoy this art of domination and submission. One of the more typical bondage positions consists of having the person being immobilized lie down, face up, with their arms extended behind them, while the master or dominant secures their hands so they can later subject their submissive lover to all kinds of pleasures and perversions.

If you want to go a bit further, you can make your partner lie face down while you bind their hands and feet behind them. This position leaves the person completely immobilized and, in the woman's case, with the vagina and anus at the mercy of any games and penetration. In fact, this is an ideal bondage position for anyone who especially enjoys anal sex and vaginal penetration from behind.

A similar option (more comfortable for the immobilized party) consists of placing the submissive person on hands and knees and binding only their arms so that they are able to move a bit more.

The best position, when it is a man who is being tied, is to sit him on a chair and bind his hands behind the chair back. This way, the other partner will be able to climb on top of him and perform some of the typical dominant positions (see page 54).

5. Swinging

Switching partners is becoming more prevalent among people who are looking for new sensations beyond what they have experienced with their regular partner.

Swingers (as practitioners are called) tend to be married couples between the ages of thirty and fifty, willing to have purely sexual relations with other married couples with the express knowledge and consent of their conjugal partner.

This is a big change to the intimate routines of any couple. Before jumping in, it is necessary to talk about it frankly and find out if the idea really is stimulating and, if both are in agreement, how best to make this fantasy, one of the most common but least practiced, a reality.

Generally, it is better to take the first step with a couple who are experienced swingers, in order to avoid possible mental blocks from both parties.

Going to a specialized club is the simplest and most direct way to meet with an experienced couple. Before crossing the threshold, you should keep in mind a few recommendations:

- Agree on the limit of how far you both want to go.
- Never lose visual contact with your partner while having intimate relations with another person.
- Be constantly asking if the other person is comfortable.
- Don't forcefully try something out that only one of the members of the couple finds attractive or exciting.
- At all times, be sure to separate the love relationship from the strictly sexual and physical one.
- Strictly follow the four rules of etiquette that accompany this kind of practice: discretion, respect, hygiene, and immediate acceptance of rejection.

Although the typical profile of swingers tends to be couples that are already together, some swingers clubs also accept men and women who are by themselves.

When trying to maintain a master/dominatrix, slave/submissive relationship with your partner, it might be exciting to "order" or "obey" when talking about switching partners with another couple. Most likely, it would have never occurred to you to do this. Now you have the ideal excuse to try it out, as part of a BDSM game.

6. Make Me Submit

Many BDSM practices have a strong and—for many—exciting component of humiliation. Facesitting is an intense twist on classic cunnilingus. The technique consists of sitting on top of a partner's face, so that the butt rests squarely on top of the submissive lover. Aside from granting the resulting pleasure to the dominant partner, the facet of domination and submission may be equally exciting for the submissive person, who may enjoy feeling trapped or immobilized between the legs of his or her partner. You can increase the intensity of this position if you tie the hands and legs of your sexual "slave."

You can choose among the different variations of facesitting depending on what appeals to or excites you at any given moment: literally sitting on your partner's face, supporting yourself or lightly sitting on top without exercising force, standing up with your partner's head between your legs, etc. Make sure you are completely in control of the pressure and your movements.

When doing this, you could surprise your partner when they are lying down (in bed, on the couch, on a lonely beach . . .). Approach them suggestively and show off your delights. You can tell them that you are burning inside and you need them to quench you with their breath. Or give them a session of oral sex and then ask if they would like you to sit on their face. Sexual relationships have a large component of mystery, so pique their curiosity and surprise your partner with something different.

This BDSM technique is also excellent for trying another game that many of you have surely fantasized about. Facesitting is perfect for enjoying an exciting session of anilingus, or the black kiss. Oral stimulation of the anus is a very pleasurable technique, since it has a great number of nerve endings, making it one of the most erogenous parts of our anatomy. It is essential to practice proper hygiene in this area and not to force the situation if there are too many qualms. There are lubricants available on the market that come in mint, chocolate, or lemon flavors that will help you to "savor" the moment. Or if you prefer, just before starting you can eat an extra-strong menthol candy or use a bit of toothpaste to mask the flavor and odor during the rimming, or black kiss, session.

7. Step Hard

One of the most simple yet BDSM techniques is called trampling. This basically consists of stepping all over your partner, either barefoot or wearing high heels. This technique particularly arouses those people who have foot or footwear fetishes. If you do this barefoot, the trampling may turn into an erotic and stimulating way of massaging your lover's body. If you do this while wearing heels, you must be extraordinarily careful not to hurt any of the more sensitive areas of the body.

Start by making your partner lie face down and naked on the floor, the couch, or the bed. Wearing only a pair of high heels or stilettos, climb onto his back and, after sensually rubbing his back and glutes against your naked skin, carefully stand up and, using the wall to keep yourself from falling down, submit your lover to a gentle and suggestive trampling session.

Another way of trampling consists of sitting on a chair and pressing your feet onto different parts of your submissive lover's body. This way, you may be able to more easily control your strength and movements.

For those who are more advanced, another technique is to place a pair of bars to the sides of your play area, or hang them from the ceiling; that will let the dominant person precisely control their movements while balancing themselves.

It is best to step on the back, the chest, or the legs, avoiding the abdominal region, the neck, or the genitalia. It's better to start barefoot, to avoid damaging your lover if you happen to slip. You should avoid unbalanced positions on top of the body, and always have something to support your weight, such as a wall. If you are wearing heels, do not apply all of your weight. Always support yourself with your toes and avoid exerting too much pressure with your heel.

8. Dressed for the Occasion

To raise the temperature of your BDSM-based sexual encounters, one of the best things to do is to wear certain articles of clothing favored by individuals who engage in this kind of sexual practice. This "dress code" usually includes latex, leather, and vinyl clothing, as well as openly fetishistic elements such as corsets, fishnet stockings and garter belts, shoes or boots with stilettos, etc. This doesn't mean that you must use all these garments. The idea is to incorporate this kind of play in the most natural way possible. Adopting a role may be a fun way of doing this. Try pretending that you don't know each other and you are in a BDSM club, for example. Let your imagination fly: maybe he is waiting for his girl and when she eventually doesn't show, he starts talking to you. You might be an experienced dominatrix who initiates the novice in sadistic practices. Wearing sensual and fetishistic items of clothing makes it much easier to sink into the story. Remember that with these kinds of games, what is seen is just as important as what is imagined.

When picking out articles of clothing, opt for what makes you feel sexier, and don't forget accessories—perfumes, makeup, etc. Dressing for sex is one of the best forms of foreplay before an unforgettable night. If you are choosing to adopt the roles of master/dominant and submissive/slave, you will be faced with very exciting choices. The person with the dominant role could order their partner to dress in a series of specific articles of clothing, and make them put them on or take them off at will. Another exciting possibility is to make a pact wherein the dominant partner will always decide when and how any future sexual encounters will happen. To make the situation even kinkier, the dominant person may have an entire closet full of clothes at their disposal that they can employ during any unexpected encounters. The thought of not knowing when or how the next sexual encounter may happen will keep the flame of curiosity burning and will be a very exciting experience.

9. You've Been Bad . . .

Has your guy behaved badly? Punish him with a few sensual lashes on the backside. Spanking is a BDSM practice that consists of striking your lover's ass using different tools. Sex shops and specialized stores carry all kinds of paddles, crops, whips, and rods that can be used to exercise an exciting and original domination/submission technique, although you may also use your hands or a rope.

To begin with, I recommend using a riding crop (such as you would find in equestrian sports) as its rigid but flexible texture is ideal for initiates. There are many models (leather, wood) with different shapes and finishes.

On the other hand, a paddle is much heavier because it is wider, and its lash will be much more intense. They can be round or rectangular, some with rivets.

If you really want to surprise your lover, get yourself a leather or latex whip. This is the lightest and most flexible spanking device, but be careful: its use requires a certain amount of mastery to avoid going overboard with the punishment.

For the most daring, there are bamboo rods. These inflict more pain than any other tool and are great for lovers of very strong sensations.

Whether you are the spanker or the spankee, remember that the goal of this practice is not to damage, but to produce an exciting submission scenario.

If you prefer, you could also dress up (as a nurse, a soldier, a boss, etc.) for a more dramatic and theatrical touch.

When spanking, remember that it is always best to do it to the backside, especially in the middle, where the body's fat will soften the blows. BDSM techniques like these are especially sensual when we employ them with a calm demeanor. I recommend going slowly and alternating between kisses and tender lashings, applying ice cubes, or covering the area with cream in order to reward their "obedience" by licking their wounds.

10. Dinner Is Served

Have you heard of nyotaimori? It is the practice of eating sashimi or sushi served on the naked body of a woman (nantanimori, in the case of a man's body). Imported from Japan, this sexual game may be a very exciting incorporation of our most intimate activities. Invite (or order, in the case of dominant/submissive role-playing) your partner to get naked and take a relaxing, perfumed bath. If one partner is in the dominant role, they can ask the other to clean and pamper them as if the two were a prince/princess and their servant. While drying, go to the kitchen and prepare everything you will need for the sensual banquet. Ask your partner to lie down on the bed and blindfold them. Take this time to bring the food to the bedroom and begin the nyotaimori session by carefully pouring a bit of sparkling white wine into their navel. To avoid any spills, you may use a small stopper or a syringe. Slurp up this frothy elixir and continue serving, on their naked skin, all the delicacies that you have prepared for the two of you. Food with a creamy consistency is best for serving directly on their body (hummus on their nipples, strawberry jam on their lips, etc.), as well as foods that can be picked up with your fingers and shared with your partner so they may also enjoy. The possibilities are endless: thin slices of smoked salmon on their abdomen, round slices of tomato on their nipples, thin pieces of carpaccio on their neck, shavings of Iberian ham on their inner thighs, rosemary honey on their pubic area, etc. It's important to make it a ritual and make sure the moment is special for the both of you. This delicious meal for two could end in a bath or shower during which you may continue living out your sexual fantasies. If you need a bit of inspiration, a director named Isabel Coixet introduced this curious erotic gastronomic practice in her film *Map of the Sounds of Tokyo,* and series such as *Sex and the City* and *CSI: NY* have also featured scenes including body sushi.

11. Trying Aphrodisiacs

They come in the form of food, condiments, body massage oils, perfume, infusions, and even incense. Natural aphrodisiacs are a natural component that should be kept in mind for your sexual relations. Sex is a pleasurable torrent of physical and mental sensations. It excites us, relaxes us, seduces us, gives us vitality, etc. It never leaves us indifferent. I invite you to try natural aphrodisiacs during your play time and experiment with your and your partner's reactions. Bit by bit, you'll discover which ones have the most sensual effect:

- **Cinnamon.** One of the most well-known aphrodisiacs. When eaten, it stimulates the heart and blood circulation, making it ideal for long, passionate nights. Try mixing powdered cinnamon with a bit of sugar and dusting your lover's body. During a make-out session, the sweet aroma and flavor will do the rest.

- **Ginger.** Stimulating and invigorating, it is perfect for revitalizing the body and gaining energy. Make a homemade massage oil by mixing oil with crushed ginger root and letting it steep for three weeks.

- **Oysters.** They stimulate the production of male hormones.

- **Mint.** Menthol oil creates an exciting, refreshing, and warm sensation, especially when applied to the genitals. In fact, gels meant to stimulate the clitoris contain menthol in their ingredients.

- **Nutmeg.** It awakens sexual appetite and can be found in spices, incenses, or in essential oils.

- **Dates.** They provide a great amount of energy and vitality. Arabs consider dates to be a sexual stimulant.

12. Burning Sessions

Nothing is hotter than a wax session. Erotic games using wax can be a very exciting innovation during sexual relations. This practice originates in the BDSM world and can be adapted to the personal taste and limits of each couple. I must insist upon the importance of being especially careful when playing this kind of game, since it can be dangerous. The key is in finding the right candles to use. Personally, I would recommend paraffin wax candles, because their wax melts at 54 degrees Celsius (129 degrees Fahrenheit) and they are better for not harming the skin. These are the classic long white candles that are often used at home, and they are cheap and safe. Under no circumstance should you use beeswax candles, because they burn at higher temperatures and you could get painful burns. And even though you might like the idea of mixing a wax session with some aromatherapy, it's not especially recommended to use perfumed candles either, because they contain chemical substances that also make them burn at a higher temperature. It would be best to go to a sex shop where you will surely find all sorts of candles made for intimate use. How should a wax session go? After lighting the candle, let it burn for a few minutes. This way, the liquid wax will build up enough that you will eventually be able to pour it on your lover's skin. This is the most important step of all. Keep in mind that the closer the candle is to their body, the more intense the sensations will be, since with a greater distance, the wax will cool before it reaches its destination. The idea is to pour the wax from a distance of approximately 20 cm (about 8 in). If you want to avoid a scare, you can test the temperature by letting a few drops of wax fall on the inside of your arm. It is also important to properly choose the areas to be stimulated. You might try drizzling wax on the abdomen or over the chest, the legs, the back, or the glutes. It's best to avoid the genitals and other sensitive parts of the body, such as the breasts, the face, etc. If you want to increase the intensity of the session even more, try blindfolding your lover so that the unexpectedness of the sensations makes them much more intense.

This game is very kinky and exciting, but it is important to be very cautious. Be sure you have your partner's consent on everything and, if possible, protect the skin with some type of cream or body oil that will make it easier to remove the wax from the surface of the skin.

13. My Slave's Collar

Imagine that one night you have your lover's body and will at your disposal. Domination and submission games can be very exciting, especially when they happen without warning.

During BDSM sessions, one partner will usually wear a metal or leather collar that symbolizes the surrender, an agreement to give themselves to a master or dominant person. Beyond the symbolism, it can also be charged with sensuality and fetishism. Nevertheless, when incorporating a submission collar into your relations, you must set some limits for the purpose of avoiding accidents. As far as using it, it could be attached to a small leash so that the submissive person is completely under the control of their master or dominant. Any game or position will be "forced" by the person assuming the dominant role, "compelling" their lover to obey their every whim. If a collar would be excessively humiliating or painful, the symbol denoting property could also be represented by a bracelet, piercing, rings, or even a small, more-or-less visible tattoo.

Those of you of a certain age will remember the *Emmanuelle* movies, erotic icons of the 1970s. Played by the Dutch actress Sylvia Kristel, Emmanuelle appeared on the posters wearing nothing but a long pearl necklace. This type of necklace is a sensual element that, besides being a very sexy and aesthetic accessory, may be used during sexual relations to increase the kinkiness and intensity of orgasms. First of all, you must choose a good one. It should be long enough (about 80 cm or 31 in) to allow you to comfortably manipulate it, and the pearls should be smooth and round (without edges or points) and secured firmly. You will also need a good lubricant that will ease the movement of the pearls across the different parts of your (and your partner's) body. For example, you can lubricate the penis well, wrap the necklace around its base, and stroke it up and down with interlaced hands. The pearls will roll up and down the length of the member, creating pleasurable and exciting sensations.

You could also use the pearl necklace to stimulate the anal region, one of the most sensitive regions that may help you experience truly intense sensations. For example, you could sensually massage your partner's glutes and anus with the aid of a good lubricant. While rubbing the area with the pearls, you might go even further and slowly introduce a small section of the necklace into the interior of the anus. Just as with Ben Wa balls, using this type of necklace will lead to some very intense orgasms if withdrawn from the anus just before climax. This game might make you a little uncomfortable at first, so you might opt for practicing it on your own at first and then, once you're used to it, incorporating it into your relations.

14. Total Control

When taking advantage of the power that a dominant lover has over their partner, there are specific sex positions that will help you to experience the most intense orgasms. Here are some ideas that you might try out with your submissive lover:

■ **The subdued.** With him lying on his back, the dominatrix will sit on his penis with her back to him. In this position, she controls the rhythm and intensity of the coitus at all times. It also allows for a special amount of anal stimulation and will guarantee very deep penetration.

■ **Tamed.** With the man sitting down, the woman sits on top of him with her back to him, letting him penetrate her from behind. This position lets the lover's hands roam wherever they want over her body in order to stimulate and stroke where he pleases.

15. My Master's Briefcase

Have you yet to try any sex toys? You don't know what you are missing. Whether you enjoy yourself alone or with a partner, the list of toys and sexual items that you could incorporate into your intimate games is quite suggestive.

One good way of jumping in is to adopt a submissive role and let your master submit you to different experiences. For example, you might act out a scene in which you receive a visit from a traveling sex toy salesman. After giving his presentation, the salesman might suggest trying out one of the items and "submit" you against your will and in your own home. You should let your imagination fly and come up with kinky scenarios that ignite the libido and help you escape your routine.

It might be hard to get used to at first, which is why it is important to choose well, so that both partners feel comfortable with this new "guest" in their most intimate relations. It is best for the couple to agree and even go to several erotic shops together in order to decide what kind of toy will be the most comfortable and exciting to begin with.

One of the best beginner's sex toys is the vibrator. There is a wide range available for purchase, including different shapes, sizes, and colors: clitoral, anal, and vaginal stimulators, double-sided, men's vibrators, etc. You can also choose among different materials such as silicone, glazed ceramic, aluminum, etc.

You can try them out without any hesitation, or use them bit by bit. One good idea might be to use it for massaging. After your normal foreplay, you could lie down naked in bed and lose yourself in a session of sensual massage with the help of a good body oil that has been warmed up. When the pivotal moment arrives, you will run the vibrator along your lover's body, exerting pressure on the back, the neck, the abdomen, the glutes, the scalp, etc. Trade the vibrator between yourselves so you can both enjoy its sensual tickling. When the temperature reaches a boiling point, you may move it to the more intimate areas. Keep in mind that some models have different speeds, which will let you adapt the speeds to the different parts of the body. Although vibrators might be known exclusively as women's toys, consider that they may also be exciting for him. They are great for stimulating areas like the anus, the perineum, or the testicles. Just remember, to avoid any sort of reluctance, you should choose a model that does not reproduce the shape of a penis too accurately.

Cock rings are also very easy to use and perfect for beginning to experiment with sex toys. They are placed around the male member with the goal of increasing blood flow to the area. Due to this, the penis swells a bit more than normal, the erection lasts longer, and the ejaculation is delayed. You can purchase cock rings made of leather or metal; some even come with a small vibrator that stimulates the woman's clitoris during penetration.

Try out some different games and let yourself get carried away.

16. Look at Me, Look at You

Dressing up and playing different roles during sexual relations activates one of the most stimulating senses: sight. Go even further by strategically placing a mirror inside the bedroom. You will have seen this in more than one movie; the typical ceiling covered in mirrors. But you should realize that in this way, only one of the two lovers will be able to enjoy the "views." If you would like to share the reflection, it would be better to opt for a standing mirror, leaning vertically against a wall, or you might even hang a mirror horizontally from the headboard.

The best position for you both to enjoy the reflection is doggy style, which is well liked by both genders, although, curiously, for different reasons. Men like it because it is a position of dominance, and women because it is a position of submission.

In this position, the woman crouches on her hands and knees with her legs slightly apart. The man gets on his knees and penetrates his partner from behind. In this position, both may look at themselves in the mirror and might even imagine that they are the other person.

Remember that the brain is the most erogenous organ we have, so let your imagination fly. You can also ask your partner to put on a mask to increase the level of kinkiness by imagining you're having sex with a "secret" lover.

17. Will You Climb on My Swing?

How many sex positions have you tried? Classic missionary, doggy style, or another? With each different position, you can experience different sensations and deeper or shallower stimulation for each partner. The idea is to learn little by little and to occasionally distance yourself from the classic positions that have become ordinary and not exciting or pleasurable.

Mainly, you should know that the woman's orgasm is much more intense when using the following sex positions:

■ **Lotus flower.** While he is sitting cross-legged, she sits astride him with her face to his. This position particularly stimulates the clitoris and the man has his hands free for stroking his partner.

■ **The tarantula.** He sits and leans back, supporting himself with his hands while his legs are stretched out in front. She sits astride him, putting her weight on her hands and legs.

■ **The horse.** During this position, the man lies face up and the woman sits on him with her back to his face and her knees on the bed. This way, the woman is able to stroke her partner's penis or her own clitoris while she is being penetrated.

■ **The other missionary.** She lies face up with one leg in the air, resting on her partner's shoulder. He stays on his knees, holding his partner's upraised leg with one hand.

■ **The spoon.** Both partners lie down and the man places himself behind his partner. In this position, almost the entirety of both bodies are in contact and the man may stroke his partner's breasts during penetration, kiss her, bite her neck, and manually stimulate her clitoris.

■ **The cowgirl.** In this woman-on-top position, she can more easily reach orgasm since the penis has easier access to the clitoris. Plus, she can better control the movements of coitus.

■ **Sideways.** Both partners lie down, face to face, while her legs "embrace" the man's body. This is the best position for making love while relaxing, allowing the couple to stroke, talk, and kiss. It is one of the more romantic ones.

■ **Reverse cowgirl.** The woman sits on top of the man with her back to him. In this position, penetration is very deep and she can control the movements at will. Plus, if you do it in front of a mirror, the woman's view will be wonderful.

■ **The crab.** She lies on her back and lifts her legs, placing them on her partner's shoulders. He places himself above her and penetrates her deeply and very pleasurably.

But don't be selfish. Keep in mind that your partner will be driven wild by other positions that, due to their angle or depth of penetration, will be much more exciting for him. Among these positions, you must try:

■ **Doggy style.** The woman gets down on her hands and knees while the man kneels or stands (if she is higher up, such as on the bed) behind her and penetrates her from behind. This position tends to be equally pleasurable for both genders.

■ **Tamed.** The man sits comfortably while the woman sits on top, facing him.

■ **The missionary.** This most traditional position is one of men's favorites. The woman lies face up with her legs open and the man penetrates her from on top. He controls the movement at all times and the view is very exciting for him.

■ **The dragonfly.** Both partners lie on their sides. He places himself behind her and she moves her leg, bent at the knee, toward her partner's back. The man penetrates the woman, using her leg, which is resting on his hip, for leverage.

If you really want to feel strong emotions using nearly impossible positions, then you should do it suspended in the air. Relax—I'm not talking about jumping with a parachute or doing it in an airplane lavatory. I'm talking about using a sex swing, known also as a sling. This is a series of padded ropes (made of leather, nylon, etc.) that are adjustable using a system of anchors that attach to the ceiling. The specialized design will allow you to rest your legs, hands, back, and butt while making love. Made for two people, it will let you try out all kinds of sex positions, some of them quite difficult to achieve without this contraption.

18. Punish Me, Darling . . .

One of the most exciting BDSM toys is called punishment clamps, and they are often used during dominant/submissive role-playing. They are designed to exert varying amounts of pressure to either a man's or a woman's nipples. This part of the anatomy is an extremely erogenous zone, and you'll be surprised by how pleasurable this can be.

There are different models, so you might want to go to a specialized shop and consult with a professional. There are adjustable clamps covered in silicone that clamp down very softly, models that come with chains attached to small metal weights that cause intense sensations when attached, vibrating clamps, and ones decorated with feathers. Keep in mind that before applying the clamps, you should stimulate the nipples by pinching them with your fingers, biting them, or applying a bit of ice so that they get hard. Generally, you shouldn't use them for more than fifteen minutes straight or they could cause pain.

As with any BDSM practice, the couple should agree upon what the acceptable limits are and decide on how intense the game should be so they can both have fun without having to be in pain. With clamps, it is especially recommended to agree on limits, since you are dealing with an extremely sensitive area.

19. Strong Emotions

This game is only recommended for daring lovers who are fond of strong emotions. The idea is to have furtive and very quick sex in an office, small storage closet, or an isolated meeting room in some public office building. You'd be surprised at the number of couples that seek out this kind of adventure in out-of-the-ordinary locations. You just need to take the plunge.

Sex at work can be very exciting but a bit risky since, if you get caught, you might be in for a bad time and even lose your job. It is still, however, a very popular fantasy, so if you want to make this dream come true, you may want to do it in someone else's office.

Convince your partner to accompany you to "pick up some paperwork" you need. To make things easier, I recommend making a visual inspection of the location days in advance in order to have the most discreet room or office in the building picked out. Try to opt for a public office building (such as a government office building, which will be full of offices, conference rooms, and people going in and out nonstop).

Once you control the "territory," head to the office building at the same time as most of the employees are greeting the arriving public.

Don't tell your partner what your true intentions are, to make the surprise even greater. Enter the office in question, lock it from the inside (choose a room where this is possible), and just start kissing him. You need to act quickly and deliberately. You should get your partner excited in record time to avoid any interruptions. It would be best if there were a good meeting table to lie down on.

And relax, because if you get caught, you'll just have to endure a moment of embarrassment and avoid being immediately fired. Your partner will surely remember that afternoon for a long, long time. Speaking about official locations, another place often frequented by couples who love furtive sex is museums. Take advantage of a Sunday morning to cultivate your intellect as well as your libido. Choose a less popular museum and, before they close, ask your partner to accompany you to the bathroom. These kinds of venues tend to keep their bathrooms very clean and they are usually in isolated, quiet areas.

20. Eat Me

A sexy way of putting your guy's condom on is by doing it with your mouth. Be careful with your teeth because you could damage the latex. This is great for men who lose their erection putting it on. To avoid this comedown, or simply to have some exciting fun, put the condom in your mouth, with the tip pointing towards your tongue. Next, wrap it around the penis and slowly, as if you were performing fellatio, push the rigid ring towards the base of the penis using your lips.

21. Tell Me . . .

Smartphones, social networks, and the Internet have all made appearances in our sexual habits. If you haven't tried using any of these things, then it's about time you did. They are a very efficient resource for seduction over long distances that can help increase the intensity of our intimate encounters.

Experimenting with more daring sexual practices tends to be a bit embarrassing or hard at first. Thankfully, phones can be an excellent medium for breaking the ice and jumping into exploring new sensations. One simple, yet exciting game consists of calling your partner on the phone (when you know they are not busy and can give you the required attention). Explain to them that you are very aroused, thinking about one of your last steamy nights. Describe to them in detail everything you remember, placing greater emphasis on what you enjoyed most. Tell them that as a reward for their efforts in bed, you want to offer them a very special gift. Don't go any further and tell them you will call them again later. The plan is to lengthen the mystery as much as possible and let your partner's imagination fly while they fantasize.

At the end of a few hours, call again and tell them that you have everything you need and to meet you tonight at a hotel. Tell them to ask for you at the reception desk and to then come up to your room. If you really want your partner to remember this date, once you're in the room, dress up in a leather or latex bodice, stilettos, and a mask. At the appointed time, leave the door to the bedroom cracked open and kneel next to the bed. When he comes in, tell him that tonight you're his slave and you'll obey every single one of his commands. He'll be so surprised that he won't know where to begin. Whisper to him everything you're willing to do for him and show him your slave carrying case, full of all the necessary toys for submitting to his will: handcuffs, ropes, crops, small whips, dildos, etc.

After this night, promise him that there will be new calls with new requests. A suggestion: Next time, you can be the dominant one and he the complacent slave.

22. Wireless Sex

The newest sensation in new sex technologies is called LovePalz. This is a device divided into two different pieces: Hera (for her) and Zeus (for him) stimulate the male and female organs in a basic way. When being used while the partners are apart, each device transmits to the other what both people are doing with their sexual organs. During this cyber-encounter, the couple just needs to connect the devices, place them on their erogenous zones, and open the phone app. Once they are connected, any movement that either person makes with their devices will be felt by the other person in real time.

23. Sexting: Look How Hot I Am!

Sexting is an up-and-coming sex practice. It consists of sending sexy messages, images, or self-recordings through cell phones. Especially popular among younger generations, this can be an exciting game to use when inviting your partner to a session of rough sex.

This practice does come with certain risks, because once you send the messages, they are out of your control and you run the risk that they may break free of your intimate sphere. So, if you are up to trying out a little sexting, try to send images in which you are not recognizable. Also, if you store this material, use a secret password that will make it hard for anyone to access that content, such as in the case of a lost or stolen phone.

Even though it may seem obvious, it is of the utmost importance to always double-check the recipient before sending so you don't send a compromising picture to your boss or parents. If you want to be overly cautious, there are apps like Snapchat that let users send pictures, messages, and videos that are deleted after a few seconds, once they have reached their destination (after ten seconds or so).

Sexting can be an exciting technological ally when tempting your partner to a night of passionate sex. Send him a recording, detailing everything you want him to do to you when he's home. Show him how excited you are by sending a cropped picture where your hand is stroking your breast or playing with your clitoris. Ask him to do the same and to surprise you with a "gift" to get your appetite up. You could even drop by a sex shop and show him some of your purchases (a whip, a latex corset, a dildo, etc.).

You can become real twenty-first-century sexters. Young people aren't the only ones doing it; even well-established couples are livening up their relationships using new forms of interpersonal communication.

24. "Oral" Sex

If words excite you, you can try phone sex by calling an erotic hot line. It is best to have a hands-free phone, so you can turn on the speaker and share the fantasy while you are doing it in bed.

The Internet can be an excellent tool for your most daring games. You can connect to a video chat and enjoy a direct feed of some pornographic sessions while you and your partner have sex. Enter terms like "web cam porn" and "cybersex" into any search engine and click on the link that most excites you.

25. Pegging: Do You Dare?

One of the most intense male submissive techniques out there is pegging, during which the woman penetrates the anus of the man with the use of a dildo that she wears using a harness. What is completely taboo for some heterosexual men may be for others so extremely pleasurable that they can experiment with even more sensations by stimulating the prostate, or the male G-spot. If your guy is reluctant, talk to him first about trying it out, because he doesn't have to go through with it.

There are several types of strap-ons for pegging, but one of the best incorporates dual pleasure, thanks to the added vibrator that is attached to the part of the strap-on in contact with the woman's vagina.

Do not skip the foreplay (stroking, kissing, etc, with the goal of dilating and relaxing the muscles around the area); it will be important to enjoy the moment of anal penetration with more intensity. It is also very important to use a good lubricant (especially for this kind of penetration) and to go slowly so that the experience is as pleasurable as possible.

This practice is exciting for many women because it flips the normal roles. They go from being penetrated to being the penetrators, from submissive to dominant.

If starting out with a strap-on seems too much for you, you can start by using special dildos made for stimulating this area, as well as beads and anal plugs, and using special lubricants that, aside from lubricating the area to be penetrated, also have slightly numbing substances.

26. Anal Pleasure

Before fully introducing this technique into your relations, you can start by lightly massaging the anal area. Ask your lover to lie face down and start massaging his whole body. Slowly approach his genitals, stroke them, play with them, make sure he is fully aroused, and only then start to stimulate the anal zone. Use plenty of massage oil and be delicate and gentle. Rub his back, whisper arousing things into his ear, and, most importantly, pay attention to his reactions at all times.

27. The Contract

During sex games with dominant and submissive roles, one element that increases the kinkiness of the relations is the existence of a contract written together by the couple. Like the contract between Grey and Anastasia in the popular trilogy by British author E. L. James, this unique and sensual document is a mutual pact that will help the dominant and submissive to lay down some rules and regulations during relations. The contract is thought of and written together, and will normally include the needs of the slave/submissive, the punishments, the rules of the master/dominant, and the signatures of both.

An example of a submission contract would look something like this:

Let this document serve to recognize my full and absolute surrender to the desires of my master/dominant, whom I accept to serve and obey whenever he/she requires my services or attention. The present contract has been written and accepted consciously and without any coercion. The articles contained within establish rules accepted by both signing parties. A failure to obey them will result in the dissolution of relations.

Article 1
As laid out in this document, I surrender myself to my master/dominant in both body and mind. Regardless of the unpleasantness that some of his/her commands may cause, I hereby promise to blindly follow and obey all of the orders, punishments, and humiliations that he/she imposes upon me, so that I may fully please him/her as his/her slave.

Article 2
The agreed-upon duration of the submission will be of seven days and seven nights, beginning from the time this contract is signed. Upon its resolution, if there is still a desire to prolong the state of submission and property, a new document will be written, in which the conditions may vary.

Article 3
In order to tame my free will, I consent to being bound and muzzled by my master/mistress and humbly accepting their commands and requirements. Similarly, I promise to please my master/mistress during any games and sexual situations that he/she imposes on me during the period of validity of the contract.

Article 4

I fervently wish to give my master/mistress the greatest amount of pleasure I can. To this end, I will dress in fetishistic clothing that will be of his/her liking and I will always be available to him/her to satisfy his/her desires by using me.

Article 5

In order to maintain my safety, both parties agree to establish a safe word (STOP) that, upon being uttered by the slave/master, will instantly halt any situation or practices that may be excessively painful or humiliating. Any situation in which this safe word is not obeyed by the master/mistress will signify a break in, and subsequent dissolution of, this contract.

Article 6

The slave/submissive is expressly forbidden from:
- Opposing the wishes or disobeying the orders of his/her master/mistress.
- Refusing the clothes, toys, or other sexual elements that he/she is subjected to by the master/mistress.
- Denying or resisting the domination by his/her master/mistress.
- Not satisfying anything specified by the previous articles.

Article 7

The slave/submissive may be marked by his/her master/mistress with a distinctive element that will symbolize his/her surrender and submission. This will be a non-permanent attribute (necklace, ring, earring, piercing) that the dominant person may flourish with pride in public as well as in private. This item will be returned upon resolution of this contract.

Article 8

The slave/submissive agrees to accept any punishment that the master/mistress wishes to inflict, whether it is deserved or not. The manner and duration of the punishment will be always to the liking of the master/mistress.

Article 9
This contract may not be altered unless both parties are in agreement.
If the conditions of these articles change, this contract must be
destroyed and a new one written and signed.

Article 10
This contract may be terminated at any time by either party.

Signature of the master/mistress　　　*Signature of slave/submissive*

28. Here and Now

In the car, on the beach, in the office, or in a hospital bathroom. The kinkiness and excitement of having sex in a public area is a truly unforgettable experience. Having wild sex doesn't just mean using sex toys or trying out impossible positions. It can also mean breaking taboos and daring to experience high-voltage situations.

For adrenaline junkies, being risky, breaking routine, and having sex in public are very common fantasies. Remember, you should always follow certain precautions if you want to avoid a bad time. If you've never tried this, you should start by doing it in a quiet area, far away from prying eyes. Remember that open areas allow for a quick retreat if needed, even if they are more exposed to unwanted visitors.

Clandestine sex could also be outlined in the submission contract if you are playing the roles of master and slave. These types of contracts (see page 67) are easy to write and they spell out the requirements and limits of the sexual games that the couple wants to play during a fixed amount of time.

Roles can change and each partner may, at any time, take up the reins and decide which sexual adventures to go on. For example, a master or mistress may command their slave to have sex in an area where they might be discovered, such as in their office bathroom or in their building's parking lot. That fear of being caught doing something forbidden will make the encounter much more exciting.

This game is excellent when rekindling the flame of passion and breaking with the routine of ordinary and predictable sex. In these cases, it's best to play around with the element of surprise. To accomplish this, you could send your partner some suggestive message or image before meeting them in a mall, using the excuse that you want them to help you pick out some sexy new lingerie. Once you are together, show them your shameless side and ask them to try out the new lingerie by making love in of the mall's public bathrooms. They won't forget that shopping trip for a long time.

29. Warming the Engines

According to a recent study by an insurance company, more than 30 percent of drivers admit to using, or having used, the car for sexual relations. This is because sex on wheels is one of the best options for a quick and kinky session of passionate sex in a public place, while running the risk of being discovered.

Leaving the bedroom and trying new places to have sex is key when it comes to breaking routine and renewing your latent passion. This change of scenery wakens the senses and will help you live out the moment with much more intensity and abandon. Besides, the car offers the added security of being able to make a quick escape if someone bothers or surprises you.

Even though improvising is great when it comes to incorporating games and fantasies into your relations, you can plan the encounter by inviting your partner along for a unique weekend. Take your car (or rent one) and hit the highway with no particular destination. What matters here is the journey, not the destination. Suggest taking a few rest stops during the trip. At each one of these stops, surprise them with a different sexual experience: oral sex, masturbation, exciting positions, etc., without leaving the car, which will be your personal love nest.

Keep in mind that the back seats have much more room for trying out different positions, although your reaction time will be cut down if you get surprised.

You can prepare a playlist to go along with your games to play on the car's stereo. Use the glove compartment to store some kinky toys (dildos, vibrators, Ben Wa balls, masks, etc.), and bring a beach cooler with a cool bottle of good white wine, etc.

As far as positions, one of the kinkier and more comfortable ones you can try in the reduced space of the car is the classic 69. The missionary position is one of the easiest to do in a car, as long as the man is not too tall. It is best to do this with the front passenger seat reclined and for the woman to make things easier by flexing her legs and placing her feet on the seat. Another kinky position you could try is to make use of the back seat so that the woman can get on all fours with her hands on the window while the man penetrates from behind. This way, the sides of the back doors can be used as support and the movements will be much more firm and intense.

If the dimensions of the car simply do not allow for great achievements, you can always exit the vehicle and use the hood as an improvised support point on which you can do some crazy things.

Another kinky wheeled fantasy you could try out is to rent a limousine with driver and do it while you drive through the city streets. You could even ask the chauffeur to park in front of your office or workplace so that every time you go to work, you have an exciting, sweet memory of the encounter. You can go online to find businesses that offer this service discreetly and seriously.

30. Very Intimate Jewelry

Small accessories are very important if you want your sexual encounters to climb in intensity. You can give your naked body a glamorous and kinky touch by using all kinds of intimate jewelry and decorations that will serve as the perfect complement for a very wild night.

Surprise your partner by adorning yourself with exotic and suggestive nipple pasties, magnetic piercings, anal beads, or suggestive penis rings. The goal is to show off your most sensual areas. You can also use accessories and sex toys that look like elegant jewels. These are a series of two-in-one pieces that are great for making some of your most sensual fantasies a reality. Some of them can be armbands that turn into handcuffs, leather and metal belts that become whips to be used during a sadistic night, necklaces with stimulating vibrators for your nipples, or adjustable bracelets for the wrist or penis that will provide more intense sensations during penetration. You may find and acquire some of these kinky accessories on www.incoqnito.com

31. To the Water!

Switch up the locations of your sexual encounters and you'll experience new sensations while you break with routine, one of a couple's greatest enemies. Have you ever tried doing it in the water? Whether it's on the beach or in a river, a Jacuzzi, or a pool, it is certainly a kinky and sexy way to make love, especially if the area is open and you might be discovered. If you feel hesitant, remember that having sex is one of the most fun things you can do, both physically as well as mentally. Letting it become monotonous and boring, or letting it blossom as what it truly is, is in your hands and in your imagination.

If you allow yourself to try out this game, before jumping into the water you should remember the following tips so that everything goes as planned:

- Even though it may seem counterintuitive, water will dry you out and can affect vaginal lubrication, making penetration harder to achieve. So keep this in mind, especially if you are in a hurry.
- Even if you've seen it done in movies, giving your partner oral sex under water is not a particularly pleasant experience. More than likely you will end up swallowing a lot of water, so it would be better to do this at the water's edge (the edge of a swimming pool is ideal).
- Water makes your bodies weigh less when you are in it, which will let you try out sex positions that require a bit more effort, such as when the man holds the woman up with his hands under her glutes while she wraps her legs around him, suspended in the air.
- If doing it in the water turns out to be a bit uncomfortable, you can always have your foreplay in the water, and then finish out of the water. The combination of both settings can also be very exciting.

32. Get Naked for Me

When it comes to extreme and daring sex, there are endless kinky and exciting games with varying levels of intensity. In many of them, humiliation is an important component, such as in the case of clothed female, naked male (CFNM). During this sexual practice, the man remains completely naked and at the mercy of the woman, who remains clothed the entire time. She is the one who controls the situation and decides what games to play for her own enjoyment.

During this game of domination, the naked man is simply an object in his partner's possession. The kinkiness can be increased by adopting suggestive roles, such as the classic doctor and her patient, an executive and her employee, a gardener and the woman of the house, or a delinquent and a policewoman.

There are different variants of CFNM that you could employ. For example, the woman could be in charge of taking off the man's clothing while slowly rubbing her hands along his most sensitive areas, torturing him with pleasure without touching him directly. Or she could ask him to get naked for her, or keep him naked around the house for an entire afternoon while he obeys her every command or whim.

Of course, these roles could be reversed and the game switched around, so that it is she who remains naked and he who is dressed. As you know, variety is pleasure.

33. Recording

Have you ever watched yourself having sex? I'm not talking about the classic reflection in the mirror, but something much more exciting and suggestive. Recording yourself on video during your intimate encounters can be an unforgettable experience. Besides enjoying the set-up and filming, the tape will later serve to help you remember those sensual moments, correct or improve positions, and of course have a good time and even get aroused and head back for a second round.

Both partners should know about the recording ahead of time, as they will be recording very intimate moments. It will require a good amount of discretion as well as a promise not to use the images outside of the couple's sphere.

Another exciting idea is to connect the video recorder to a television in the same room and enjoy a direct feed of all of your intimate and loving endeavors.

For the most daring of you, the recording could be uploaded to some free porn website so you can share your adventures through the web. Many people will see it, since this type of material is currently the most downloaded porn on the Internet.

One way or another, you should enjoy the entire process of recording, by choosing a well-decorated stage, imagining a story or an everyday situation to act out, being mindful of the lighting and avoiding shadows, getting yourselves ready, and making use of some toys or accessories, such as a sexy dress, some high heels, a latex corset, or a mask if you don't wish to be recognized.

If at first you feel a bit of trepidation or you don't know how to act naturally, you can begin with a relaxing massage and draw out the foreplay to allow yourself to forget about the camera. Putting on a bit of sensual music may also help you out.

34. Shall We Meet?

This will seem particularly daring and even risky, but it is also becoming more and more common. Initially, dogging was a practice from the United Kingdom that consisted of having public sexual relations with strangers whom you contacted through specific forums, dedicated to the practice, that take it very seriously. With the passage of time and the success of this exciting practice, meetings are held now in private homes, parking lots, sex shops, and other locales. With the goal of getting to know one another better, there are communities that count on thousands of affiliates in different cities all over the world. Registered users can arrange meetings through two systems: using the forum to arrange a public meeting, or using private messages to arrange a private or invite-only meeting.

Users share erotic and sexual photographs with the rest of the community. These show off their qualities and attributes to the rest of the community, so that, in many cases, they may be appreciated and invited to private events.

If you prefer swinging (see page 44), you can specifically seek out those kinds of anonymous encounters and later share your experiences. This is one way of enriching your sex life and learning some new techniques at the same time. When engaging in these types of practices, you must practice safe sex and always use condoms.

35. In a Hairy

Sometimes a simple change can give your relations an exciting new touch. I suggest taking a look at intimate hair removal. Comfortable, attractive, and hygienic, shaven genital regions will allow you to experience more intense sensations during penetration because there is more contact with your naked skin. And it goes without saying that if you tend to practice oral sex, you will always be grateful for a lack of hair, which you may choke on and ruin the magic of the moment.

When erasing the hair from your intimate areas, you have a few choices.

- **Normal shave.** This is the classic removal of hair that we all know, where you only remove the hair in the groin area.
- **Brazilian shave.** Consists of removing hair from the pubis, without going as far as the lips.
- **Caribbean shave.** Completely removing the hair from the entire pubic area.

For men, the process is similar, and they can shave the hair from just the groin or from the entire pubic area, including the testicles.

Along with hair removal, and if you want to give your intimate areas an aesthetic touch as well, you can try out some intimate decorations. This means creating curious shapes with your hair, and even using different-colored dyes. There are centers that specialize in decorating the pubic area and can shave you in the shape of a heart, star, triangle, etc., and even dye you pink, yellow, blue, etc.

As a couple's outing, getting your genitals shaved can be a fun and sensual experience. You could prepare a relaxing, foaming hot bath, letting the steam and water soak into your skin. After a while, sit on the edge of the tub with your legs open, watching your partner, who is still in the water. Then, your lover may begin applying abundant amounts of soap to your private area (Editor's Note: be careful to only use a soap that you're comfortable with) and start cutting off your pubic hair with the aid of a pair of blunt-tipped scissors. Because the skin in this area is extremely sensitive, it is best not to do this in a hurry. Next, it is the other person's turn. You should switch positions and continue with the ritual without forgetting to end by applying a good amount of hydrating cream to the recently shaven area to avoid any irritation.

36. The Box of Desires

Keeping the flame of sexual desire burning in a couple who has been together for a long time requires imagination, creativity, and daring when incorporating new experiences into the relationship. Sex games can be the best antidote for fixing routine, apathy, and even boredom in bed. Imagine that you eat the same thing every day; you'd end up getting bored, right? Well it's exactly the same when it comes to sex. You need to use new ingredients and seasonings all the time in order to fully enjoy and savor your sexuality.

The idea behind this is very clear, although sometimes it's not as easy to put it into practice. When you've been together a long time, you tend to take a lot of things for granted and believe that you know each other's sexuality completely. It's as if there are no more secrets or mysteries between you, and you come dangerously close to becoming conforming, routine, and predictable, like many other couples. It is up to you to switch gears. It is perfectly normal to feel inhibited, or a bit shameful, when first sharing your sexual fantasies and desires. But keep in mind that your partner is not a mind reader, and cannot guess what it is that you wish to change or add to your sexual relations. The change begins by starting to communicate what your preferences and sexual fantasies are, and what you would like to try or experiment with. Many people don't take this important first step for fear that their partners will take it the wrong way and feel guilty for the current situation. Keeping quiet is not the answer, I can assure you. Mind you, it is important to communicate your desire to improve your sexuality with a bit of tact if you want to avoid hurting your lover's feelings. Try to frame the topic positively: "Honey, I love living with you. You take care of me, make me smile, spoil me, and excite me. Do you know what gets me excited?"

In this manner you can introduce the topic of sex and at the same time find out how much your partner knows about your sexual preferences. Don't let them change the topic on you. Ask them question after question about their likes and sexual fantasies, what they would like to try, or what is missing from your intimate relations. Most importantly, this is a time to be sincere, uninhibited, and to let the imagination fly. The key is in getting both partners to better know how to excite, attract, and light the flame of desire of the other. That key will open the doorway to new and exciting experiences, and you will only be able to enter it through dialogue, imagination, and a bit of daring.

One simple and fun way of sharing your secrets is to use a box of desires. The idea is simple: you each buy a pretty little box and write down, on five colorful little papers, five games or sexual fantasies that you would like to try as a couple. This is not the time to be shy. Take all the time you need; think about intimate experiences that you find exciting, daring, fun, and unique. Once these suggestive boxes have been filled, decide who will start the game. Once a week, without letting the other know, one of you will open the other's box and fulfill their wish or sexual fantasy until all the papers have been taken out. The box of desires will help you break the ice, incite your sexual initiative, and encourage you to try new and sensual sexual experiences.

If you want to go a bit further, I suggest you try a more intense variant. This variant is the master's/mistress's box. When you do this, the dominant partner will put five commands into the box that their slave/submissive must comply with to satisfy them. In this book you'll find all kinds of ideas and possibilities that you can try out.

On a different occasion, you can switch roles and the dominant can become the submissive. This game will definitely be fun.

37. Sex Is an Affair for Two . . . or Three

One of the most common sexual fantasies is to have a threesome (either with two men and one woman, or two women and one man). Usually, this idea is brought up by one member of the couple. Thus, it is important that the other partner be sure that the idea pleases them and does not make them feel embarrassed or rejected.

With this kind of practice, there need to be previously agreed-upon conditions, such as the role that each partner will adopt (active lover, voyeur, etc.), who will be the third person, what kinds of things will be allowed or not (anal sex, vaginal penetration, etc.), what things you would like to share only with your partner, what implications this will have for your sexual relationship, etc. The decision to form a threesome needs to be understood, accepted, and agreed upon by both. You might even entertain the possibility of adding a fourth person, turning it into a swinging situation (see page 44).

Once you have made up your minds, the next step is to find someone interested in a threesome. Social networks and online forums are great for tracking down candidates.

Once you've found the right person, you should arrange a meeting in a neutral place. There are hotels that exist exclusively to facilitate sexual encounters that will provide you the necessary amount of privacy.

If it's your first time, it makes sense that you will feel nervous and tense. Break the ice by having a nice glass of wine while you talk a bit and share your preferences, tastes, and intimate desires. Make sure you center the conversation on sex from the start, and avoid topics having to do with work, family, or offspring. You'll find that, little by little, the situation will start to heat up and slowly turn to stroking and kissing. Keep in mind that in games like this, it's important that everyone feels comfortable and nobody feels left out.

If the threesome is composed of two women and one man, some exciting things to try could be for one woman to perform fellatio on the man while the other woman sits on his face while he gives her cunnilingus, or for the man to masturbate both women at the same time. If they are especially daring, one of the women could use a strap-on and penetrate the other, or even anally penetrate the man.

If the threesome is composed of two men and one woman, she can give both men oral sex at the same time, experience the intense pleasure of double penetration, or perform fellatio on one of them while the other penetrates her from behind.

Your imagination is the limit.

38. A Tantric Night

A few months ago, I ran into Eva, an old friend. She was totally radiant. When I asked her what her secret was, she confessed that it had to do with tantric sex. Ever since she started practicing it, everything was going better with her partner, they had recovered forgotten sensations, and she felt closer to her guy than ever. As I was in a bit of a hurry, I invited her to have dinner with me that night at my home so we could talk more. I didn't want to miss that!

Eva came with her boyfriend Stephane who, like her, looked spectacular. During the meal they explained to me that they had been about to split up until a friend invited them to spend a long weekend in a rural home. This was not a hotel; this was a place where men and women gathered to take residential courses and where many couples came to initiate themselves in tantric sex.

"A place of presence, fun, pleasure, spirituality, and discovery," Stephane commented while piercing my eyes with his deep gaze. That man was truly attractive, and for a moment, I let my imagination take me away. Maybe the wine was to blame, or maybe it was the presence of that man talking about tantric massages, but I suddenly started to notice a warm tingling that made me sigh. My guests gave each other a mischievous look and Eva asked me if I would like to try everything that they had learned. She knew that I was always ready to try out new things. Stephane's hand softly stroking my knee had made up my mind for me. We turned the lights off and I lit a few candles and turned on some relaxing music. The three of us sat on the rug and started to stroke each other and gently take each other's hands. Little by little, my mind entered a state of complete relaxation while I focused all my attention on the sensations of my skin. The stroking started getting more intense, until Eva's hands began to take off my clothes. Stephane took my hands and invited me to do the same thing. With my eyes barely open, I took off each item of his clothing until we were naked from the waist up.

The ritual advanced slowly, while we listened to our own breathing, giving all our attention to the reactions of our bodies. That sensory complicity was truly pleasurable, but my physical side fought to speed up the process. I was very excited and could feel my heart beating strongly beneath my naked and erect breasts. It seemed that Stephane caught me blushing because he started kissing me slowly, first along the length of my neck and moving down until I could feel his hot breath between my breasts.

Eva did the same thing to her guy in a sort of synchronized dance of suggestive, harmonic, and sensual movements. I think we must have been like that for over an hour, feeling each movement, each brush, each look, each kiss, and each stroke. "Would you like to try the asanas of love?" Eva whispered in my ear. Stephane remained completely naked and sat on the rug with his legs crossed. He took me by the hand and asked me to sit on top of him with my legs open. While not once looking away, he gently caressed my glutes while delicately penetrating me. My body immediately started moving with a certain intensity, but Eva grasped my back lovingly to stop my pushing. "Gently, gently . . ." she said, while Stephane whispered to me to listen to his breathing and try to synchronize it with mine. We remained in that position of gentle balance for more than half an hour until I couldn't hold it in any longer and I had one of the most intense orgasms I can ever remember having. Curiously, this was the slowest, gentlest coitus I've ever had, but with a really explosive climax.

After that date, Eva and Stephane invited me to spend a weekend in that famous rural house where everything had started. There, I learned the importance that breathing and conscious thought have in tantric sex, different techniques for delaying climax, the art of stroking and massage, and the use of meditation to make the mind control the body during sex.

If you would like to know more about the different positions and exercises for practicing this sacred art from India, I suggest reading some books on the subject, such as *The Art of Tantra*, by Guillermo Ferrara.

39. The Foolproof Weapon

I won't be telling you anything you don't know if I say that men are driven wild by women's breasts. I remember during one of my workshops for advanced techniques to drive a man wild in bed, Rita, one of my assistants, confessed that her partner could reach orgasm just by touching them.

We also enjoy that fascination, which makes us feel sensual and wanted. However, that devotion may cause our partners to put their weight on them, bite them, or hold them too strongly. As with all the games I outline in this book, it's important to communicate to your partner at all times what you like and dislike during your intimate relations. Personally, I love it when my lover strokes the area under my breasts or runs the tip of their tongue along the outside of my areolas. On the other hand, my friend Jessica likes it when her man softly pinches her nipples and roughly kneads her breasts. The important thing is to enjoy giving and receiving what we most enjoy without prejudices or clichés. What is excessive or painful for me might be really exciting for another woman.

What is clear is that a woman's breasts are a foolproof "weapon" for getting a man aroused in record time. Does he like massages? Tie him to the bed, take your clothes off, apply perfumed oil over his whole body, and massage him with your breasts until he begs you to let him go. If you're mischievous or have a sweet tooth, put some cream or chocolate on your nipples and let him enjoy a sensual banquet without using his hands. Afterwards, you can do the same thing with different parts of his body.

Remember that there are specific sex positions that will provide more intense stimulation to the breasts. One of my favorites is domination, because it allows me to take the initiative and my lover's hands are free to massage my whole body, which is something I find especially exciting. I love the feeling of hands running all over my skin and stimulating the most sensitive areas! When I use this position, I like to make my lover sit on a chair or on the edge of the bed. I place myself on top of him with my back facing him, and I can move at my leisure, and set the rhythm and depth of penetration while he massages my back, glutes, breasts, etc.

Another of my favorite positions is the modified missionary, which I especially like on days when I'm in the mood for some rough sex. It's very simple: I lie face up and lift a leg up and place it on my partner's shoulder. To get more comfortable, I place a pillow just below my hips. Meanwhile, he will be on his knees, lifting and holding my leg with one hand. In this position, his penis fully stimulates my G-spot because it easily reaches the back face of the uterus. Try it out and you'll like it too. Trust me, I'm an expert. This position also has an element of submissiveness that gives the man complete control of the rhythm and motions of penetration, which might increase the kinkiness for him.

40. Cover Your Legs

During different workshops, talks, and conferences I've given in the United States and Europe, I've found that stockings are one of the accessories that men of all ages find the most exciting. And it's not just them. Many women (and I count myself among them) enjoy showing off a pair of sexy stockings along with some high heels. They make us feel very feminine and sexy! Suggestive to the touch and sight, my favorite stockings for sex games are made of latex or vinyl, colored black, red, or transparent. Their texture makes them feel like a second skin and this gives them an added level of kinkiness.

Place the tip of your foot on the bed with your leg bent at a right angle. Slide the stocking down smoothly until you take it off. Spectacular.

We don't like . . .

This brief section is mandatory reading for all the men who have made it this far. My purpose isn't to hurt your feelings or undervalue your efforts. But communication is one of the key aspects of every sexual relationship, so here are some things that bother most of us women, especially when we're having sex with you:

- **Lack of imagination.** There are infinite possibilities you can explore beyond the missionary position and a bit of oral sex. Why don't you take some time to explore new territory every once in a while?

- **Quiet sex.** Don't be afraid to look silly; most of us love to hear loud exclamations and insinuations. You can also let your feelings take the reins by moaning, yelling, sighing, etc.

- **Skipping foreplay.** A rushed and hurried coitus may be fun and exciting every once in a while, but what we really want is to enjoy the journey without obsessing over penetration and orgasm. Kisses, strokes, massages, role-playing, some small toys sometimes . . .

41. Free Your Imagination

Many women think that fantasizing about sex with other men (or women) is the same as being unfaithful to their partners, and they feel guilty. Remember that thoughts are not actions and neither is imagination. To become reality, fantasies must stop being fantasies. When that happens, most of the time they'll end up losing their erotic power.

I sincerely believe that most of us have fantasized about situations outside of our relationship, which is actually very exciting, so why fool ourselves? It's said that men are more likely to do this than we are, although a recent study published by *The Journal of Sex Research* under Dr. Thomas V. Hicks at the University of Vermont confirmed that eight out of every ten women have sexual fantasies about other men. Fantasizing about sex is a pleasurable and unlimited resource that can be used at any time to experience pleasurable sensations, whether we are alone or—why not?—with company.

Rose, a member of my workshop-organizing team, confessed to me a little while ago that she likes to imagine that she is being consensually raped by the attractive director of her bank when she is making love to her husband. It is a spontaneous and brief fantasy that happens every once in a while and helps her to be more active and daring during sexual games with her partner. My friend ended up confessing this to her husband, and he smiled and confessed that he, too, sometimes fantasized about the teller at the very same bank. That same night they both decided to each adopt the role that most aroused the other and they had a very intense sexual session, with BDSM games and a bit of domination as well.

It's good to incorporate sexual fantasies about situations outside the relationship into new games and experiences. The secret is to live them naturally and avoid feelings of guilt, myths, and taboos. Remember, sex is for having fun and there are no limits. By repressing this kind of fantasy, we will only manage to fall into routine and monotony, the worst enemies of a relationship. Move forward and dare to try new experiences, sensations, desires, and feelings that are socially forbidden or disapproved of. Sexual fantasies can be used to express our sexual desires and feelings, escape from real life, increase or initiate sexual arousal—both alone and as a couple—get rid of tension, or rehearse sexual behaviors that you've never had a chance to put into practice.

Our thoughts broadly influence our sexual relationships. For example, when something is worrying me, or I've had a tense day, nothing will boost my libido—not even an army of sweaty, well-built soldiers bent on satisfying my every intimate desire. I can assure you that my fantasies are most effective, but when my mind is somewhere else, there's just no way. Other times, I just need a little push to get my engine started. That's when I will use some wandering thoughts to stimulate myself. For example, I can imagine that someone is watching us through the window, or that we're doing it in a public place and someone could catch us, or that I'm with someone in particular (someone I know, a famous person, someone from the neighborhood, etc.), or that I'm being forced to have sex with someone I don't know whom I do not want.

Have you ever asked what the most common fantasies are among men? Many like to imagine they are dominating a woman through consensual rape and, though they might not admit to it, many enjoy fantasizing about being used by a transvestite or transsexual.

42. A Sensual Piercing

I'm not a huge fan of piercings, but I recognize that it can be very exciting when someone with one of those small metal balls in their tongue gives you a session of oral sex. The piercing fad goes beyond simple aesthetics. When placed on certain parts of our body, they can become an excellent instrument for increasing sexual pleasure.

Piercings can also be used to stimulate the genitals, especially the clitoris. Most women get them on their labia minora or majora, or at the base of the vaginal entrance and the perineum. These are very sensual, and playing with them can be very pleasurable.

You need to be careful when using different positions in order to avoid accidents and, as far as hygiene is concerned, to avoid infection.

Some of the most daring places to get a piercing are the nipples, the tongue (very exciting when giving your guy fellatio), or the clitoris. A belly-button piercing is less aggressive and very erotic.

If you get a piercing on your tongue, the sensations your lover receives during oral sex will be multiplied. Because it is metallic, the piercing is an excellent heat conductor and it will prove a good tool for intensifying and varying the stimulation you impart during an oral sex session. A good idea is to drink a hot or cold beverage just before placing your mouth on your partner's vulva or penis. The piercing will be the same temperature as the drink and it will be much more sensual an experience for your lover.

Make sure you go to a professional piercer and that the level of hygiene of their shop is high enough to satisfy even a dentist, in order to avoid infection or illnesses like hepatitis or AIDS.

These small pieces of jewelry should be kept clean at all times. Wash them with hot water and neutral soap after each session (avoid soap that is too strong or perfumed).

43. You're Welcome

Many people find it less than enjoyable to perform oral sex on their partner. They don't like the smell or flavor of genitals and they avoid one of the most exciting and fun sexual practices out there. To get over this dislike, I propose a romantic and exciting shared bath. You can make it even more seductive by adding some rose petals, aromatic candles, essential oils, and bath salts.

If flavor still proves to be a problem, there are endless lubricants on the market that are specially made to cover it up. They are completely edible and they come in different pleasant flavors like strawberry, lemon, mint, chocolate, and more. You can also eat an extra-strong mint while you suck on his penis (your guy will feel some very strong sensations too), or place an edible sexual lubricant capsule into your mouth and open it with your teeth while you give oral. Another option is to put a little bit of toothpaste in your mouth (for a cool sensation) or even a shot of cognac (for a warm sensation).

We were all told not to play with our food. But on this occasion, we'll skip this sage advice and turn our food into the perfect seasoning for enjoying an exciting oral sex session. Ingredients such as cream, marmalade, honey, yogurt, chocolate, and wine will let you "savor" your lover's body.

Here are some delicious recipes:

- Pour a small trickle of sparkling rosé on your lover's mons pubis. Let the small, sparkling drizzle run down her vagina while your tongue moves to meet it. Lick her lips, her clitoris, and drink the sparkling wine from the most sensual glass you can think of.
- Heat up some thick chocolate, let it cool a little bit in a bowl, and add several spoonfuls of cream. Using a brush, spread the sweet ambrosia over the belly button and genitals of your lover. Use your greedy tongue to take in the sweet banquet. Slurp, lick, suck, and devour it with pleasure.
- Mix some strawberry yogurt with a bit of honey. Let it chill in the fridge and use it to season her clitoris. Spread it gently and in small amounts. Let it slide down her hood and labia minora. You should do it very slowly so that the cold stimulates the area before you lap it up greedily.

■ Cool his penis with a bit of mint. Rinse your mouth using the most concentrated mouthwash you can find, or place an extra-strong mint candy in your mouth, and give your partner a refreshing round of fellatio. Your "mentholated" tongue will make him feel cool sensations because of mint's vasoconstrictive properties.

Don't forget to keep a box of moist and perfumed towelettes in your room so you can clean each other up after your banquet.

44. The Forbidden Zone

The anus is a very erogenous zone, but many couples have certain qualms about including it in oral sex sessions. For men, the proximity to the prostate makes it an extremely pleasurable area if you know how to stimulate it well. But keep in mind that this is a delicate subject and many men feel that their manhood will suffer if they let themselves be manipulated there.

During foreplay, you can start by giving him a gentle massage around the anus with your moist fingertips. Play with this area for a while while you stroke his testicles with your other hand. The motions should be smooth and natural, not forced at all. Ask him every once in a while if he likes it, and if he is excited by what you're doing. His moans, movements, and words will let you know if you should keep forging ahead or switch to a different area. If your guy is enjoying your efforts, start inserting your finger into his anus little by little, moving it in slow, careful circles. Any practice involving the anus requires hygiene, both for your hands and his rear.

If you want, you can also insert your hot and hard tongue into him by parting his glutes to make way, while you use another hand to stimulate his penis.

The black kiss, or anilingus (oral stimulation of the anus), is an exciting complement to fellatio or cunnilingus. It's best to get on all fours and let your partner place themselves behind you with their head beneath the arch of your legs. This way, they can stimulate and lick the entire genital and anal area, as well as play with your glutes and the inside of your thighs.

Normally, the rectal area responds to stimuli by contracting. Because of this, it's important that you let your partner relax and feel comfortable with your anal explorations before you bury your tongue in their anus. Massage their back and glutes, and kiss and stroke their upper thighs. Lick, suck, and nibble carefully on their backside, perineum, and the skin around their rectum. Lubricate and warm the area with your mouth.

The rectum will contract while it is stimulated and then it will expand. Lick or touch the rectum with the tip of your tongue, and wait for their response. Afterwards, the sphincter muscles will start to relax, allowing for a deeper exploration.

Using your fingers to provide anal stimulation can also be very exciting. The vagina shares a wall with the rectum, meaning that they also share a series of erogenous zones and very sensitive nerve endings. So you can alternate your licking and kissing with some manual stimulation (very softly, mind you, and only when the area is sufficiently excited and dilated). To do this, moisten or lubricate a finger and start to stroke the anal opening. Little by little, and very carefully, insert it until you hit the G-spot. Stimulate the area using small circular motions and by moving your finger up and down.

One last piece of advice. You need to take certain precautions when orally stimulating the anus. You need to keep in mind the presence of certain bacteria that live in the large intestine and colon, which can cause infections. If you wish to try out the black kiss, be thorough with your hygiene and be comfortable with the person you're doing it with.

45. Submissive Fellatio

I assure you that this method of having oral sex is most men's favorite, since it lets them move pleasurably and from a prime point of view, with their lover at their feet. In this position, the man remains upright with his legs spread wide open and his arms waiting to receive his lover. She can begin by stroking, kissing, and licking his neck, chest, and nipples, moving downward towards his abdomen and belly button. Meanwhile, her hands can run over his glutes, thighs, etc. The man remains standing, waiting for his lover to approach with her warm lips and give him an arousing round of fellatio.

After this foreplay, she kneels down with her face at the height of the man's pubis. She exhales suggestively onto this area while she plays with his testicles, without moving her hands away from his glutes and thighs. One of her hands firmly grips the base of the penis and introduces it slowly into her mouth. Now, there will be a series of movements that mirror those of coitus while her tongue stimulates his glans. With her lips in the shape of an "O," she surrounds the tip and frenulum of his penis and moves around in circles.

Keep his penis wet with saliva and let him feel the warmth of your breath at all times. And don't forget the other senses. Lift your gaze and look at him with eyes full of desire, and let a few growls of pleasure slip out.

This position can be very active for the partner as well, since they can hold their lover's head and direct their movements as they please. Be careful when this happens, though. In this position, men can get very excited and, while standing, start making the same movements in the mouth of their partner as in coitus. By not controlling the depth of the oral "penetration," the woman can easily choke.

In another variation of this posture, the man stays on his feet, but with his backside resting on a table, a chair, the edge of the bed, etc. She sits on the ground (or, better yet, on a pillow or cushion), sideways with her weight on one of her glutes and her knees bent. In this position, she can start playing with her lover's testicles while she firmly grasps the base of his penis. Her lips and tongue warmly stroke the entire surface of the foreskin and glans. While salivating profusely, she places his penis in her mouth and starts moving back and forth—gently at first, slowly, and then increasing the speed of the rhythm until he melts with pleasure.

If your lover feels that you are enjoying yourself while you give him fellatio, you will have already gotten halfway to the final climax. Thus, it's important that you liven up the situation. Don't skimp on the moans, the little grunts, and the dirty talk, which will all increase your guy's libido. If he sees that you are enjoying the moment, he'll get much more excited.

46. The Warrior's Rest

Rough sex and BDSM sessions are very exciting, but you should not abuse them by using them time after time, without fail. Personally, I would recommend alternating these sessions with softer sessions that will let you gather your strength while experiencing pleasurable sensations in a more relaxed setting.

I propose having a night of erotic massage, one of the most exciting forms of foreplay. It will relax your muscles, release your tension, calm your mind, and prepare you to abandon yourself to a new session of great sex. This is the time for tenderness, affection, and direct skin-on-skin contact. Caresses are the most important part of foreplay.

Erotic massage techniques require calm and the patience to wait for the right moment. Rushing is your worst enemy. It's best to have some tranquility without fear of being interrupted. Turn off your cell phone, make sure the bedroom will be at an adequate temperature the whole time (about 25 degrees C, or

77 degrees F), and put on some soothing, sensual music, and light some candles, or incense.

Aromatic massage oils and lotions will be your best allies. You'll find a wide variety to choose from on the market, but you should make sure they are all quick-absorbing. Keep in mind that creams take longer to be absorbed by the skin and they can have an unpleasant taste if you decide that once the massage is over, you want to stimulate your partner's body with your tongue or lips. Try using pure oils like olive oil, almond oil, or sunflower oil that you can apply directly to the skin or mix with essential oils like sandalwood, ylang ylang, patchouli, etc. If you prefer a homemade massage oil, you can add a couple of drops of essential oil to 30 mg (about six teaspoons) of any base oil. For mixtures, odorless oils are usually better. Forget about typical virgin olive oil because it smells too strong and doesn't mix well with the essential oils. Besides, you can never really cover up the smell with something else.

Start by undressing your partner or asking them to do it themselves. Then they should lie face down, with their head sideways and their arms bent a little bit, at head height. It is important that they feel comfortable at all times. Cover their backside with a soft towel if they are feeling cold in the beginning (the plan is to get them hot very quickly).

Warm a bit of aromatic oil with your hands (don't apply it directly to their skin because it tends to be pretty cold). Slide your soaked fingertips along the skin of their back, trying the following motions:

- **Circular.** Use the palms of your hands to rub their back in different ways, in a clockwise direction.

- **Sliding.** Place your hands on the base of their back, with your fingers pointing towards their head. Using your body's weight, slide both hands up the length of their spine.

When performing erotic massage, you can stroke and gently rub their extremities, their hands, their feet, and their face. Try out a gentle head massage as well. Pay special attention to the temples, the crown, and the back of the head. This area is extremely sensitive and your partner will melt with pleasure.

Bit by bit, you'll get deeper into the back, the neck, the shoulders, and the legs. The next step is to stimulate the thighs, the groin, the chest, and lastly the genitals.

Remember that this doesn't just consist of rubbing the skin with your hands; you can also use objects like feathers, tassels, silk handkerchiefs, etc.

Many areas are sensitive to soft stroking, such as the earlobes, the cheeks, the neck, the back of the neck, the Adam's apple, the inside of the arms, the belly button, the calves, and between the fingers and toes.

You can also use saliva and gentle breaths of air to vary the temperature of certain areas of skin, such as the back and the neck.

Enjoy the sensations of your partner's body during the erotic massage, such as the feel of their curves, the tension of their muscles, their shape, and the contact with their naked skin. Appreciate each detail and express your passion and affection.

47. Online Inspiration

The Internet is an excellent tool for awakening one's libido. There are innumerable pages where you can download all kinds of free videos. If you are lacking inspiration, I can assure you that the Internet is brimming with stories, positions, scenarios, techniques, etc. A piece of advice: If you want to watch longer X-rated videos without having to play two or three in a row, you should search using the type of category you want—mature, lesbian, MILF, amateur—followed by the term "tube." You will see a huge number of results with specific videos of varying lengths (between five minutes and an hour) on the theme you chose.

48. A Different Kind of Masturbation

Feet are frequently forgotten during sexual relations. This despite its being one of the most fetishistic parts of the female body. We can incorporate feet into our intimate games in different ways.

Besides dressing your feet up in high heels, fishnet stockings, latex, or vinyl, you can surprise your guy with a foot job. This kinky and arousing technique consists of masturbating the man using only your feet. It's essential to keep your feet well taken care of, with clean nails and hydrated skin, so that contact with your partner's penis is as pleasurable as possible. You can also dress them up with some suggestive stockings or even stimulate him with your high heels on, although you should wait until you are a little more experienced before attempting this unique masturbatory art.

I remember that the first time I tried a foot job with my partner, it was a complete disaster. I could not find a position that was comfortable at all and I felt like my legs were too heavy, so I gave up (although I compensated him in other ways). After several attempts, I found that the best position for doing this requires both partners to lie on their backs and for the woman to lie in front, with her knees bent like a butterfly and her feet together. From there, the idea is to place the bottoms of her feet around the penis and to move them up and down. To make things easier, I apply a good amount of hydrating cream or oil to the area to make sure my feet can move with ease.

Another simple foot job position involves sitting on a surface above your lover, such as if your guy lies on the ground while you sit on the couch. This way, you'll have more control over the movements, although your legs might end up feeling very heavy.

If you think you can't do it on your own, just ask your guy to help you by holding your feet and moving them how he wants.

49. A Burlesque Night

A couple of years ago, I was invited to the premiere of a burlesque show. For those who don't know, this is a type of theatrical piece from the eighteenth and nineteenth centuries, normally acted out by women dressed garishly, exuberantly, and sensually. They were very popular in Parisian cabarets at the time and, little by little, fell into obscurity until their aesthetic made a recent comeback in the world of movies, fashion, music, and literature.

I confess that during the trip, I became more and more excited while watching the kinkily, provocatively, and sensually dressed women. I didn't delay in surprising my partner with a burlesque look that left him breathless. Since I know that pronounced curves are my strong point, I dressed in a well-adjusted corset that sensually lifted my breasts and hips.

The four spots

■ **G-spot.** The Gräfenberg spot, or G-spot, is a small area inside the female genitalia, located behind the pubic bone and around the urethra. Imagine the face of a clock with its center located in the vaginal opening. If 12 o'clock is facing the belly button, the G-spot is located between 12 and 1. To find it, insert two fingers into the vagina (ring and middle fingers). Keep them arched and make a tapping movement (not a penetrating one). Do it rhythmically and constantly. For this technique to be most effective, make sure your hands are totally clean, with trimmed nails. You couldn't go wrong with a bit of cream or massage oil if your hands need to be smoother. Keep your fingers inserted in the vagina. Imagine that there is a sort of egg resting partially on the back wall. Gently surround the egg, stroking it with your fingers. If you notice a more swollen area, you've found the G-spot.

➤

- **A-spot.** Located in the front of the vagina, about 2-3 cm (3/4-1 in) before getting to the uterine collar and a bit after the G-spot. To stimulate it, you should slide your fingers halfway along the top of the back vaginal wall. There you will find a larger area, a bit rougher than the regular vaginal wall. This is the A-spot. Stimulating it is practically the same as stimulating the G-spot, and doing so will help you achieve multiple orgasms (if you are well lubricated).

- **K-spot.** Located at the end of the vagina, almost at the neck of the uterus. You can only stimulate it through penetration, because the penis needs to enter deep into the vagina. The ideal position to do this in is with the man facing the woman, who is lying face up with her legs on his shoulders.

- **U-spot.** An area very close to the urethra, just under the clitoris. It is very pleasurable when stimulated orally. To do this, apply some strong and constant pressure to the urethral area with the lower lip and teeth while orally stimulating everywhere else using the tongue. One could also separate the labia minora to completely uncover the urethral area and stroke it gently with the tongue.

Plus, I put on some fishnet stockings, gloves long enough to reach my elbows, some frilled short shorts, and 20 cm (8 in) heels. I decorated my naked breasts with a pair of pasties (nipple covers) with leather tassels that I moved suggestively from side to side. Covered in a feather shawl, I waited for my guy to come home while lying in bed next to an ice bucket with French champagne, a small whip, and my little bag of intimate toys. The rest of the story, I'm sure you can imagine.

50. Sweet Veneration

I love to discover new sex games! One of the latest I've tried is sexual worshipping or veneration. The practice consists of concentrating on one sole sexual organ for the longest time possible, saturating it with sensations until reaching orgasm. Related to oral sex, this is one of the most intense forms of foreplay, so much so that it may even make penetration unnecessary.

The penis, testicles, anus, clitoris, G-spot, and breasts all tend to be sensitive erogenous zones perfect for playing this game. The plan is to make your partner completely relaxed and become completely passive. To help them concentrate for a long time, you can prepare a relaxing environment, put on a little music, light some candles, etc.

Once the stage is set for your game, you will begin to manually and orally stimulate only the erogenous area you've chosen, using gentles caresses and licks. Remember that the key to worshipping is in the rhythm of the game, so it's important that you start off slowly, without rushing, to prolong the stimulation as much as possible. You should try to avoid having the other person reach climax immediately so that they are focused for at least fifteen minutes on the one area without getting carried away. During stimulation, it's good for your lover to tell you everything they like or dislike the most so you can adapt the worshipping. Remember, during longer periods of sexual activity, it's best to use plenty of cream or lubricating oil (edible, if you are having oral sex).

51. Non-Consensual Sex

The success of E. L. James's trilogy has caused one of many women's most frequent, yet hidden, sexual fantasies to surface. Role-playing a rape, or non-consensual sex, with varying degrees of applied force and domination, is a sex game that requires a certain amount of interpretive abilities to adopt the roles of the aggressor and the victim, but it is extremely pleasurable for many couples. On the surface, this might seem like an unpleasant re-creation of something that unfortunately happens for real, but the key lies in being able to separate reality from fiction, and being able to imagine the desire to be "punished" for being "too sexy." This is fiction that you can act out using all kinds of sex toys, handcuffs, gags, tape, ropes, ski masks, etc. to make the story more real and exciting. By the way, do you know about ball gags? This sex toy is well known among bondage and domination fans. It consists of a ball, usually plastic, that is placed in the mouth of the slave/submissive like a gag, in order to keep them from speaking and submitting them to the master/mistress's will. This rough sex toy tends to be used in role-playing scenes involving rape or kidnapping. Since you are using an object that restricts breathing and prevents the gagged person from talking, you must substitute a clear game-stopping gesture for your safe word (snapping fingers, a well-placed strike with the hand, etc.). You can find all kinds of ball gags in specialized sex shops, some with very suggestive designs, but there are other simple alternatives, such as using a long piece of cloth or a rope that you can run through the mouth and tie at the back of the head.

Just as with other domination and BDSM practices, before trying out this kind of game, you must agree on a safe word or gesture that will allow you to instantly put a halt to the activities if either of you is feeling uncomfortable. It would also be good to remember that this sort of recreation can grab neighbors' attention if you are not discreet enough. If you would like to avoid a visit from the police about your interpretive theatrics, you might want to be discreet with the thumps and screams that you'll be making.

52. Lovers with a Sweet Tooth

Sex and food are two great pleasures, although they may cause totally different reactions in our bodies. Enjoying both of them at the same time is an experience that no one should miss; a delicious feast for sensual gourmets. The ancients already experienced both kinds, as we can see in the *Kama Sutra*.

During this game, all you need are sprinkles, those tiny little pieces of candy that decorate baked goods, cakes, donuts, cupcakes, pies, and ice cream. Give your lover a nice surprise and start by smearing your lips with a little bit of honey. Next, add the chocolate or caramel sprinkles. The sweet nectar will make sure they give you their attention for a good long time, ensuring that your lover will be able to taste your sweet gift without any haste. Next, take off your partner's clothes and pick out a spot on their body to decorate with sprinkles. You can create entertaining shapes, words, messages, or arrows that point toward a specific part of the body. Alternate roles so that both of you can enjoy eating and being eaten. This game can have endless possibilities for oral sex. If you can't find sprinkles, a simpler, yet just as tasty, alternative is grated coconut, ground almonds, or sugar.

If you like the idea of decorating and devouring your lover's body, you can also try out some edible body paint. Using this suggestive form of foreplay, you can turn your naked bodies into sensual canvases upon which you can unleash your artistic inspiration. You should exchange your usual sheets for an older set, or cover the bed with a bedspread or blanket that you don't need, so you can forget about possible stains. This is an excellent opportunity to tell your partner how you feel by writing messages on their skin, or guessing what pictures are supposed to be. You could even write down sex games that you don't dare speak of, as a way of inviting your partner to try them out. To answer your invitation, the other person can use a different color to respond. For example, if they draw a red line, it could mean "don't cross," or if they draw a green circle, it will mean "go ahead." Don't forget to bring out the camera to immortalize the sensual memory of this artistic night. You could even use an instant camera to suggestively decorate the room.

53. Chilling

The skin is an especially erogenous zone that responds intensely to all types of stimuli: kisses, pinches, tickles, strokes, etc. It is also very sensitive to changes in temperature, a reaction that you can include in your sexual games. For example, a sensation of cold will cause the skin to become much more sensitive to stimuli. Thus, it can be fun and exciting to use ice cubes during your foreplay, especially during a hot summer night. Slowly take off your partner's clothes and slowly rub their skin so their body starts increasing its temperature. Take your time, stimulate their most erogenous zones, add a brief period of oral sex, and when you see that they can't take any more, put an ice cube in your mouth and run it along their burning skin. Run it down their neck, around their chest, and down their abdomen to their belly button. Stop there and let it fill with water. Slurp up the contents, tickling their skin with the tip of your tongue. Suck the ice cube back up and descend down their legs until you get to the bottom of their feet, between their toes. Repeat this process on their back; descend towards their glutes and the backs of their legs. Don't hurry, and let the stimulating contact with the ice cover your lover's skin in sensations.

When your partner can't take it any longer, warm their spirits up again by caressing, kissing, and massaging them with your naked body. Get them turned on again and then move on to the second course. Cover different parts of their body with sweet and creamy ice cream. Savor it naughtily by licking, sucking, and slurping it all down to the last drop.

54. This Is Good for . . .

Imagine that there are pieces of paper with writing on them hidden all around the house, and when you find them, you can trade them for sexual activities. Don't tell me that doesn't sound exciting! The surprise or tension that exists before sex is almost as pleasurable as the act itself. Besides, the idea couldn't be simpler. All you have to do is cut out a few pieces of paper (if you want, you can decorate or color-code each one by the level of intensity), write down the sexual activity, and hide them around the house (inside a closet, among your underwear, behind the mirror, etc.). Agree with your partner beforehand how far you are willing to go with the written activities and if you are ready to enjoy them without qualms. For hiding places, it's better to choose two or three simple spots so that the game can start immediately, and then place the rest into more hidden spots to draw out the mystery as much as possible.

The rules of the game allow for two possibilities: the simpler of the two is that each person writes the coupons for what they will do themselves. This way, they will be in complete control of the situation, but it will also reduce the element of surprise. The other option is for each partner to write down what they will be looking for, and so the other partner won't know ahead of time what they'll be doing. This game is perfect for breaking up sexual monotony, and it's ideal for experiencing new sensations in a playful and casual manner.

55. Please, Go On!

Let me suggest a sweet and suggestive domination game for torturing your partner. You will be in absolute control, so tell your lover that they can go crazy. He'll be the protagonist of this soirée, but at no time should he disobey the rule of not interfering. Don't reveal any more of the mystery, and let his imagination do the rest. Remember that sexual tension is one of the kinkier and more exciting facets of intimate relations.

Start as soon as you can so that his curiosity doesn't flag. Take him to the bedroom and ask him to slowly and unhurriedly disrobe. Don't approach the bed yet. Place yourself behind your lover and start whispering sensual (and dirty, why not?) things into his ear. Tell him how much a certain part of his anatomy excites you, or everything you're going to do to him so that he melts with pleasure and begs you to end this torture. At no time should you touch your lover while you talk to him; let his sexual tension start gaining heat.

Now you get naked too, and start running your finger (or a small feather) along his body, gently blow on his skin, nibble him, kiss him, and lick him on different parts of his body, but never approaching any of his erogenous zones. The idea is to lightly increase his libido without completely turning it on.

Continue the sweet torture by inviting your lover to bed. To make his submission absolute, you can handcuff him to the headboard, tie his hands with a silk handkerchief, or cover his eyes with a blindfold. Depriving him of one of his senses will make the experience more intense. Using a good body oil, start massaging him from the waist up. But don't do it with your hands; use your body to sensually stroke his skin. It's imperative that you continue without approaching his most erogenous area, no matter how much he begs you. Remember that you're holding the reins tonight. If you use an edible body oil, you can run your tongue along his body, kiss him, or bite him. Don't forget sensitive areas like the nape of the neck, the neck, the ears, the lips, and the inside of the arms. Keep going down and start slowly stimulating his thighs, approaching his genitals, but never going as far as touching them. Go back up until you reach his abdomen, letting your hot breath stimulate his secret area on the way, but not touching it. Softly caress his chest, kiss it, nibble it, and moisten it with your tongue. The key of this game lies in stimulating him in intense, but very short, bursts. The continual interruptions to his pleasure will make this pleasant torture more and more unbearable. By now, his body will be very sensitive to even the lightest stimulation. Take advantage of this heightened arousal to give all your attention now to his genitals. It's time to present him with a well-deserved oral sex session and finally untie him to end the sweet torture.

56. A Good Ally

To be able to fully make the best of your nights of great sex, it's imperative that you have a good headboard. When trying out certain sex positions, you'll need a solid area to support yourself on comfortably that will let you place yourself in different positions so the stimulation can be deeper, kinkier, and smoother. It should be strong enough to bear the brunt of your passionate activities and, hopefully, solid enough to keep from banging against the wall due to your movements (or the neighbors will be calling at your door).

If the structure is not pleasant, or if it has sharp edges that could cause bothersome scrapes, you could try covering it or draping it with some sort of cloth, or try to make do with some soft, XXL-sized cushions. I know a few couples that, in addition to their headboard, have bars anchored into their walls so they can hold on to something firmly, without being afraid of breaking the structure of the bed. This could prove effective if you have an excessively old or fragile headboard.

Besides being there for support, you can use your headboard to handcuff or tie up your partner during intimate domination games, like bondage. Depending on its structure, it could be used to store all the tools and toys that you want to keep close at hand (such as body oil, dildos, vibrators, gags, Ben Wa balls, condoms, etc.).

57. Can I Have Your Belt?

Something as simple and apparently harmless as a belt can be an excellent tool when breathing new life into your sexual games.

The belt is an article of clothing with a lot of possibilities when trying out bondage and other domination and submission techniques. Wide or narrow; cloth or leather; with clasps, buckles, tacks; the shape is what matters least. What really matters is letting your imagination loose, digging it out of your drawer, and leaving it on your nightstand or wrapped around your headboard so that you have it at hand whenever you want to break with the routine of your intimate encounters.

Belts are of utmost importance during games that involve spanking, when you can fold the belt in half and use it to strike your lover's backside. More than the pain itself, this kind of game focuses on the kinkiness of punishing a lover, forcing them to follow your orders, and submitting them to your will. Just lightly hit your lover's backside, and you'll succeed in generating a satisfying sound that will quickly get you in the mood. You can add to this game by creating a scenario (e.g., an elegant medieval lady punishing the stable boy, an emperor making his slave submit to him, etc.) in which you can employ all kinds of gentle and kinky punishments. In fact, just threateningly holding a belt is already an element of domination, so you can use it without ever needing to actually strike your partner.

Another kinky way to incorporate the belt into your sex games is to use it as a leash or collar for domination. You just have to run it through the buckle without securing it, so that it tightens when you pull on it. You can use it to make your partner submit, putting it around their neck and forcing them to do what you want through small, dominating gestures or tugs on the belt. It's important that you not let yourself be taken away by the passion. Control the pressure of the punishment at all times so that you don't cause painful welts or suffocate your partner.

A safer yet equally exciting option is to use the belt to immobilize the hands or feet of your partner and try out some of the kinkier bondage sex positions that I suggest on page 43.

The belt, like many other leather or plastic articles of clothing, has an exciting fetishistic facet to it. You can use it as an aesthetic accompaniment to an erotic show or a striptease, as well as during foreplay, along with other items such as masks, gloves, or high-heeled shoes.

58. Fortune Cookies

During my workshops and conferences on sexuality, many people have described difficulties in trying to suggest new sexual activities to their partners. Because of shyness, a fear of being rejected, or insecurities, they end up blocking their desires to experience new sensations and staying immersed in their sexual routine. I always recommend breaking that barrier through communication and, if it is still too hard to express their fantasies, I suggest that they use sex games that incorporate small written messages.

For example, a few simple fortune cookies can be turned into the perfect precursor to spending an unforgettable intimate night together. Each partner writes five short messages detailing some game or sexual fantasy that they would like to try. To begin, choose easy things, like a sensual massage, a new position, or oral sex in the shower. To maintain the element of surprise, each partner should keep their messages secret until they appear inside the cookie.

Another option is to write the messages together and decide between the two of you which games you want to try.

It's important to choose the right time to open the cookies. It's best to do it at the end of a relaxing date, kind of like a sensual dessert, and fulfill each wish one by one, without rushing and enjoying the ritual. Making fortune cookies can be a lot of work. The best thing is to take it slowly and dedicate all the time you need. Remember that the sexual tension can be very great, so you can turn the culinary experience into a whole other sex game. Leave your clothes in the bedroom and cover your body with just an apron. Play with different ingredients in the kitchen. The point is to savor (not devour) the whole process in order to have a very intensely enjoyable afternoon. Sometimes it's hard to let your imagination run free. You start to hurry and you have your mind on a thousand other things that block your more playful, daring, and creative side. Good foreplay is the best ingredient for savoring each subsequent moment and not letting yourself get carried away by the frenzied pace you're used to having on a daily basis. If you learn to enjoy it as it should be, your sex life will be much more intense and fun.

Here is a recipe for making ten fortune cookies. You will need:

- *The whites from two large eggs*
- *1/2 teaspoon of vanilla extract*
- *1/2 teaspoon of almond extract*
- *3 tablespoons of olive oil*
- *8 tablespoons of wheat flour*
- *1 1/2 teaspoons of cornstarch*
- *1/4 teaspoon of salt*
- *8 tablespoons of granulated sugar*
- *3 teaspoons of water*

Start by writing the messages on twenty pieces of paper about 8 x 1.5 cm (about 3 x 0.5 in). Next, preheat the oven to a temperature of 150 degrees C (300 degrees F) and prepare a sheet pan by oiling it to prevent the cookies from sticking. In a bowl, mix egg whites, vanilla extract, almond extract, and oil. In another bowl, mix flour, cornstarch, salt, and sugar. Add both mixtures together and stir well until you have the consistency of a uniform paste. Next, pour small amounts of mixture onto the pan, forming circles about 10 cm (about 4 in) in diameter, leaving about 5 cm (2 in) of space in between each cookie so they don't stick to each other. Bake for fifteen minutes, or until they turn golden. Take the cookies out of the oven and, before they get hard and you can't shape them, place a cookie on the palm of your hand (with a mitt on so you don't burn yourself), put one of the written pieces of paper on the center of the cookie, and close it, forming a half moon shape and squeezing the edges so that it seals. Repeat this process with the rest of the cookies and let them cool.

59. By the Hair

When was the last time you really let yourself go with your lover? I'm talking about losing control and letting out that irrational side that we all have hidden in a safe place deep inside ourselves. Sex, in its wildest form, can be extremely exciting. Surely you've grabbed your partner by the hair during penetration, or given them a good yank when you let yourself go for a moment. These simple gestures turn physical contact into something much more intense and kinky. In fact, grabbing and pulling hair is one of the most common practices during domination and submission games. For technique, it's best to firmly grasp your partner's hair and keep yourself in place. Otherwise, if you are pulling and letting go, all you'll achieve is pain. Either way, the scalp is a sensitive area and you would do better to start bit by bit to see if you like or dislike the experience. Taking advantage of a passionate moment, you can briefly grab your partner by the hair, without pulling on it. If after a few seconds you don't see or hear any objections, you can slowly start to pull and observe their reaction. This way, you can intensify the gesture bit by bit until the pulling is much more pronounced. In any case, always make sure to grab a good amount of hair. The more hair you grab, the more the tension will spread out among the individual hairs and the less damage you'll do. On the other hand, if you grab just a bit of hair, you could easily rip it out during a moment of passion. If your partner has a good amount of hair, you would do best to grab the hair at the back and avoid the bangs or the sides, where the pulling will be more painful. It's best to up the intensity bit by bit over time, avoid rough movements, and be careful with objects like bracelets and rings that can tangle in the hair and cause unwanted jerking. Since this is a domination game, it would be much more exciting to combine it with other BDSM games, such as a bondage position (see page 43), whipping, etc.

If you would rather not feel any pain, you can try gentler versions of the same game. It can be very sensual to run your fingers through your partner's hair while you caress their scalp, lace your fingers into their hair and then remove them gently with small tugs, or grab their head firmly while you force them to stimulate you orally.

60. Facefuck: Pure Domination

Combining oral sex with domination could be a very exciting thing to try, don't you think? This is the essence of facefucking, a sexual activity in which one lover holds their head still while the other makes penetration motions in their mouth.

This domination technique is very kinky and tends to be combined with other gestures like hair pulling, bondage, and the use of blindfolds or masks. The person who has complete control during this game is the one receiving oral stimulation, which can be switched around as the night goes on so that both partners can enjoy playing the dominating role. The submissive person doesn't have to be completely passive the whole time. The position used during facefucking (usually lying down or on their knees) will give the person access to different parts of their lover's body. They can caress or squeeze their partner's backside, play with their testicles, stimulate them anally, or even masturbate themselves at the same time.

61. Bare Your Teeth

Did you know that in the erotic traditions of India, biting is a very important element? The *Kama Sutra* gives us a good list of bites with a great deal of detail.

According to this timeless text, the areas that are most susceptible to biting are the same places that we kiss, except for extra-sensitive areas like the inside of the mouth and the eyes. You can bite almost all parts of the body. These range from a playful and harmless nibble to the strong biting that usually happens during a passionate climax. Many people avoid this last kind of biting, because it is difficult to control and usually leaves noticeable marks. Also, during orgasm, the jaw can spasm suddenly and clench down with a lot of force, which can cause injury or marks that are hard to hide. Some specific types of bites:

- **The biting of the boar.** The markings left on the skin are several lines of pronounced markings, very close to each other, with red intervals (like the footprints left behind by wild boars in the mud). This is a bite that is usually done on the shoulder.

- **The broken cloud.** This is a series of uneven welts in a circular pattern on the skin, caused by the spacing between the teeth. The *Kama Sutra* specifies that this type of bite should be done to the chest.

■ **Hidden bite.** This is the kind of bite that leaves an intense red marking and should be done on the lower lip.

■ **Swollen bite.** When you bite down on a great amount of skin.

■ **The point.** When you bite down on a small amount of skin with your teeth, so that the only mark left behind is a red point.

■ **The line of points.** When that small bit of skin is bitten with all your teeth and they each leave their mark.

■ **The coral and the jewel.** This is the bite that results from using your lips and teeth together. The lips are the coral and the teeth are the jewel.

62. Endless Torture

This domination game requires a healthy amount of self-control, but it can be very exciting and fun. The idea is to give your lover a daily session of sex using all kinds of kinky games, but without letting them orgasm until the very last day. To achieve this, you should avoid penetration or other forms of oral sex and masturbation. Throughout this book, you will find dozens of games that you can use on your lover so that by the end of their sensual torture, they are begging for release. To make it even kinkier, you can tie your partner up during the games to make sure they obey all of your commands. If they don't, you can punish them by extending the torture for a few more days.

> ## Myths be gone!
>
> Too often, the worst enemy of sexual desire is taboos and false myths that end up sabotaging our libido—convictions that keep us from fully enjoying our intimate ➤

➤

relations. We must get rid of these myths as soon as we can. Here are some of the most common ones:

- **Women who openly enjoy sexual relations are slutty or trampy.** Let's start with the most damaging and self-sabotaging myth. Free your instincts and experience your sexuality to its fullest, no matter what people around you think. They have the same sexual needs that you, I, or the rest of the world have.

- **Having sexual fantasies is something only deviants do.** The limit to sexual relationships lies in your own imagination; don't place barriers around your desire, and let your mind free itself. It's the most erogenous organ you have.

- **Every sexual relation should end with coitus.** Another common mistake. An intimate relation can be fully enjoyed without the need for penetration. There are endless erotic games (this book is full of them) that don't require coitus.

- **When a woman needs sex toys, it's because she isn't satisfied with her partner.** Sex toys are an accompaniment, never a replacement for your partner. Incorporating them into your relations is highly recommended for finding new sensations and stimuli, whether you're alone or with a partner.

- **Practices like fetishism, sadomasochism, and bondage are a perversion.** As long as these practices are fully consented to by both members of the couple, they are an excellent way of adding new games to your sexual relations.

- **Size matters.** Remember this motto: quality matters more than quantity.

63. Let's Do 69

As its name visually indicates, 69 allows each lover to stimulate their partner's genitals comfortably and, best of all, simultaneously.

This position is fairly versatile because not only can you perform simultaneous oral sex (fellatio and cunnilingus), you can alternate it with masturbatory techniques performed on the genitals or even anal stimulation as well.

Generally, the woman gets on top of the man with her genitals over his face and her mouth on his penis (if the man is on top, it's more complicated for the woman to stimulate the erect penis).

But there is a position in which both of you will be much more relaxed. It consists of both of you lying down next to each other, stretched out, with your heads next to your partner's privates.

Sixty-nine is a very exciting position, but there are a few downsides to keep in mind. On one hand, when each lover is orally stimulated, they can tend to "zone out" because of the pleasure they're feeling. This can cause either member of the pair to "forget" to stimulate the other member as they deserve. One variant of 69 that avoids this involves remaining in the inverted position but, while one partner orally stimulates the partner, the other masturbates them and then they switch roles. This way, it will be much easier for both to reach orgasm. An expert's tips: From the 69 position are born other numbers like 696, in the case of a threesome, or 6969, when you are dealing with an orgy. Another exciting variation of the position is known as 70 (or 69 + 1). In this case, the extra number is the finger that one of the lovers inserts into their partner's anus.

64. Let's Play!

Erotic table games are an excellent way to have fun while you raise the heat between you and your partner. You can go to any sex shop and find different kinds of games of varying intensity to play in pairs or in groups. These are perfect for playing during one of those dull Sunday afternoons to liven up the atmosphere.

However, I would recommend holding off until you have done some warming up first. The things suggested in these games require a lack of inhibition and it's best to bring them out after a session of kisses or massage. Just when the foreplay starts to pick up the pace, bring out the game and plan for the sexual encounter to move forward with more fun and originality.

If you prefer the classics, you can play the best bingo game of your life. Agree on a sexual activity for some of the balls: if eight, then fellatio; if fifteen, then cunnilingus; if one, a simple kiss; if twenty-five, the Ben Wa balls; and if you get bingo, then whatever you want! Another great classic is strip poker. You only need a deck of cards, a table, and something to drink. The game begins, and you make bets according to the rules. Agree on how many rounds you need to lose before starting to take off some clothes. When one of you is completely naked, then the time has come to trade clothes for actions (a French kiss, a foot massage, cunnilingus, etc.).

65. Lap Dance: Melt Him with Pleasure

We've all seen movie or television scenes featuring a lap dance. It is a sensual dance that is done on your partner's lap, imitating the movements of penetration while you take your clothes off, bit by bit, until you are completely naked.

This game is very exciting, but it requires a bit of preparation if you want it to succeed. To start with, it's important to choose the right music. If this is your first lap dance, you should opt for a sensual song with a slower rhythm so that you let your movements be slower and much more precise.

Once you've picked out your playlist, the next step is to choose a suggestive outfit that is easy to remove while dancing. Don't forget to add accessories like gloves, feather boas, masks, etc., as well as tight clothes that show off your sexiest curves.

A few days before delighting your partner, you should rehearse the dance in front of a mirror and find out which movements make you feel the most comfortable and sexy. Stop to think about what excites your partner the most, or which parts of your body get them the most aroused. If you are lacking in inspiration, don't hesitate to consult a professional and load up one of the infinite number of lap dance videos available on the Internet.

As soon as you feel ready, pick a day when you'll both be relaxed and peaceful at home, and then turn on the action. Get the music ready and ask your lover to sit on a chair. Make it kinkier and cover their eyes while you get dressed for the spectacle. Turn on your music and approach them from behind. Sensually caress their hair and untie the blindfold covering their eyes. Start the suggestive dance and make it clear from the start that they cannot touch you. Start with movements that don't involve physical contact so that the atmosphere heats up bit by bit. Next, sit down on their lap and move your hips up and down and side to side. Bring your mouth and breasts to their face, but don't let them touch. Step back if they try to touch you. If you need to, give them a few lashes or pull their hair a bit until they become obedient.

The game has an infinite number of choices: lick their lips, let your glutes brush against their chest, and drop down until you are sitting directly on their lap. Place one foot on their knees and masturbate in front of them, stick your breasts in their face, kneel down between their legs and give them oral stimulation, or finish by sitting on top of them and finally let them penetrate you.

Glossary

■ **BDSM.** Acronym formed from the initials of four extreme and nonconventional sexual practices: bondage, discipline and domination, submission and sadism, and masochism.

■ **Ball gag.** A gag that consists of a ball secured by a leather collar. It keeps the mouth open and prevents any possibility of choking because of a lack of air.

■ **Bondage.** Sexual practice based on tying the partner up, either for erotic and aesthetic reasons, or as part of a domination/submission relationship.

■ **Clothed female naked male.** During this sexual practice, the man remains completely naked and at the mercy of the woman, who remains clothed at all times.

■ **Collar.** A leather strap that goes around the slave's neck.

■ **Dirty talk.** Using rude and lustful words or phrases during sexual relations.

■ **Discipline.** Nonconventional sexual practice that consists of imposing a series of behavioral rules and executing punishments if they are broken.

■ **Dogging.** Having sexual relations in public places, usually anonymously and without any personal connections.

■ **Domination.** Behaviors, habits, and sexual practices centered on consensual relations that imply the domination of one individual by another.

■ **Dress code.** Rules imposed within a BDSM relationship in which each member of the pair must dress according to a set of pre-established themes: medical, uniforms, police, latex or leather fetishism, etc.

■ **Facefuck.** Sexual activity in which one lover holds their head still while the other makes penetration movements in their mouth.

■ **Facesitting.** Sexual practice that consists of sitting on a person's face (front- or backward facing) to force oral-genital or oral-anal contact.

■ **Fetishism.** An adoration that people profess toward a part of the body, clothing, practices, or fetishes.

■ **Footjob.** Fetishism practice of adoring feet, shoes, and heels, as well as the attainment of an orgasm by using or watching them.

■ **Lap dance.** Sensual dance that is done on a partner's lap, imitating the movements of penetration.

■ **Masochism.** Receiving intense stimulation, either physical or mental, with or without pain.

■ **Master/mistress.** Person who adopts the role of owner or proprietor of a slave.

- **Nantanimori.** Practice of eating sashimi or sushi off a man's body.

- **Nyotaimori.** Practice of eating sashimi or sushi off a woman's body.

- **Pegging.** Sexual practice in which a woman penetrates the anus of a man with a dildo that she wears using a harness or in her own vagina.

- **Rimming.** Oral stimulation of the anus.

- **Sadism.** Obtaining sexual pleasure by performing acts of cruelty or domination.

- **Safe word.** A word that is agreed upon before a session and that signifies that all actions being done to the slave should immediately stop.

- **Sexting.** Sending erotic or pornographic contents using a cell phone.

- **Slave.** Person of whom the master/mistress has ownership rights in BDSM relations. During the fantasy, each person adopts a sexual identity; this is generally temporary and lasts only as long as the bondage and submission games persist, without any implications in real life.

- **Sling.** Piece of leather, usually rectangular, that hangs from the ceiling (or a strong frame) using chains or belts. Used for comfortably being in different sexual positions incorporating penetration.

- **Spanking.** Striking a person's backside, either with one's hands or using a rope, rod, or whip.

- **SSC.** Acronym formed from the words Safe, Sane, and Consensual. It refers to the ideal model that all BDSM-related practices should follow.

- **Submissive.** Person who assumes the role of slave or servant in a BDSM relationship, and who enjoys being dominated.

- **Swinging.** Sexual practice based around exchanging partners.

- **Switch.** Person who enjoys the roles of both domination and submission.

- **Trampling.** Sexual BDSM practice that consists of stepping or walking on someone's body, with or without shoes.

- **Vanilla.** BDSM jargon that refers to those people who exclusively practice conventional sex, with no intention of trying new games or sensations.

- **Waxing.** Using the hot wax or paraffin of a candle on a person's skin to obtain sexual pleasure.

- **Worshipping.** Concentrating on one sole sexual organ for the longest time possible, saturating it with sensation until reaching orgasm.